The University of Texas
M. D. Anderson Symposium on Fundamental Cancer Research

Volume 39

CRITICAL MOLECULAR DETERMINANTS OF CARCINOGENESIS

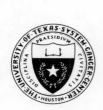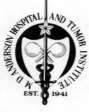

Published for
The University of Texas System Cancer Center
M. D. Anderson Hospital and Tumor Institute, Houston, Texas
by the University of Texas Press, Austin

The University of Texas
M. D. Anderson Symposium on Fundamental Cancer Research

VOLUME 39

Critical Molecular Determinants
of Carcinogenesis

Edited by

Frederick F. Becker, M.D.

and

Thomas J. Slaga, Ph.D.

University of Texas Press, Austin

Department of Scientific Publications

UT M. D. Anderson Hospital and Tumor Institute

Monograph Editors
CAROL A. KAKALEC
LORE M. FELDMAN

Copyright © 1987 by The University of Texas System Cancer Center
All rights reserved
Printed in the United States of America

First Edition, 1987

Requests for permission to reproduce material from this work should be sent
to Permissions, University of Texas Press, Box 7819, Austin, Texas 78713-7819.

Library of Congress Cataloging-in-Publication Data
Symposium of Fundamental Cancer Research (39th : 1986 :
    Houston, Tex.)
    Critical molecular determinants of carcinogenesis.

    (The University of Texas M. D. Anderson Symposium on
Fundamental Cancer Research ; v. 39)
    "Compilation of the proceedings of the University of
Texas M. D. Anderson Hospital and Tumor Institute at
Houston's Thirty-ninth Symposium on Fundamental Cancer
Research, held 16–19 September 1986, in Houston, Texas"—
T.p. verso.
    "Published for the University of Texas System Cancer
Center, M. D. Anderson Hospital and Tumor Institute,
Houston, Texas"—P. facing t.p.

    Includes bibliographies and index.
    1. Carcinogenesis—Congresses.   2. Cancer—Genetic
aspects—Congresses.   3. Pathology, Molecular—Congresses.
I. Becker, Frederick F.   II. Slaga, Thomas J.   III. M. D.
Anderson Hospital and Tumor Institute.   IV. Title.
V. Series: UT M. D. Anderson Symposium on Fundamental
Cancer Research (Series) ; v. 39.   [DNLM: 1. Carcinogens
—congresses.   2. Cell Transformation, Neoplastic—
congresses.   3. Oncogenes—congresses.
W3 SY5177 39th 1986c / QZ 202 S9893 1986c]
RC268.5.S936   1986   616.99'4071   87-10758
ISBN 0-292-71102-6

This volume is a compilation of the proceedings of The University of Texas M. D. Anderson Hospital and Tumor Institute at Houston's Thirty-ninth Symposium on Fundamental Cancer Research, held 16–19 September 1986, in Houston, Texas.
    The material contained in this volume was submitted as previously unpublished material,
except in instances in which credit has been given to the source from which some of the
illustrative material was derived.
    Great care has been taken to maintain the accuracy of the information contained in the
volume; however, the editorial staff, The University of Texas, and the University of Texas
Press cannot be held responsible for errors or for any consequences arising from the use of
the information contained herein.

Contents

Preface

In his summary of the 1986 Symposium on Fundamental Cancer Research, Dr. Henry Pitot pointed out that although it is possible to treat cancer with varying degrees of success, we still do not understand all of the molecular events leading up to its transformation and uniquely distinguishing the cancer cell from its normal counterpart. This statement gives rise to two questions at the heart of understanding the malignant process in living cells, how does a cancer cell differ from its normal cell of origin and how does a cancer cell develop from a normal cell.

The chapters of this monograph demonstrate the authors' motivation to discover the answers to these questions, and their research projects center around understanding the cancer cell in molecular terms. This volume is the proceedings of a meeting that was designed to provide a forum for the exchange of ideas and results of the mechanisms that influence the induction of cancer by chemical agents. The studies reflected in these chapters are aimed at identifying obligate interactions between activated metabolites and chemical components of the cells; the biologic alterations that result; and modifying factors, such as genetic predisposition. Specifically, the authors discussed the genetic makeup of the target cell in terms of its susceptibility to carcinogens, the expression of oncogenes, and the role of exogenous agents in carcinogenesis. One session of the meeting was devoted to discussing intracellular signals that control normal cell functions and that may deviate under the influence of oncogenes or other factors.

FREDERICK F. BECKER
THOMAS J. SLAGA

Acknowledgments

The editors would like to thank the many individuals who unselfishly provided advice and assistance at every stage during the planning and execution of the symposium. We thank the external advisory committee, Drs. David Baltimore, J. Michael Bishop, Philip Leder, Peter C. Nowell, Henry Pitot, and Stuart H. Yuspa. We also thank the session chairmen Drs. David Baltimore, Grady F. Saunders, Stuart H. Yuspa, and I. Bernard Weinstein for their guidance during the meeting.

We are especially grateful for the cosponsorship of the National Cancer Institute and the American Cancer Society, Texas Division, Inc. In addition, we extend our appreciation for the generous support of Merrell Dow Research Institute, Smith Kline & French Laboratories, Schering Laboratories, E. I. DuPont De Nemours & Company, and Hoefer Scientific.

We owe special thanks to Mr. Jeff Rasco, Ms. Shirley Roy, and the staff of UT M. D. Anderson Hospital Conference Services for providing assistance throughout the symposium and to the Department of Public Information and Education for its assistance to us and the professional and public media.

THE CARCINOGENIC PROCESS

Symposium on Fundamental Cancer Research, Vol. 39.

1. Cellular and Molecular Mechanisms of Carcinogenesis in Lining Epithelia

Stuart H. Yuspa

Laboratory of Cellular Carcinogenesis and Tumor Promotion,
National Cancer Institute, Bethesda, Maryland 20892

Lining epithelia are the major target sites for cancer in man. The induction of carcinomas on mouse skin following the application of chemical agents is the prototype model for cancer development in a lining epithelium. In this tissue, the earliest carcinogen-induced lesion, initiation, results in an epidermal cell with an altered program of terminal differentiation. Such "initiated" cells can be selected in culture since normal cells can be induced to terminally differentiate by Ca^{2+} or phorbol ester tumor promoters and will be lost from the cultured population. In situ, the growth of initiated cells is suppressed by surrounding normal cells. The differentiation-inducing effects of tumor promoters on normal cells, therefore, are essential in providing a selective growth advantage which results in the clonal selection of initiated cells and the evolution of a papilloma. This benign tumor is the pathological manifestation of the initiated phenotype. The c-ras^H gene appears to be one target for initiating carcinogens, as a mutated and activated form of this gene is frequently isolated from chemically induced papillomas. Furthermore, the introduction of an activated ras^H gene into cultured normal keratinocytes produces papillomas when the cells are transplanted as a skin graft in vivo.

After a long latency period, some papillomas convert to carcinomas. Since the conversion process can be accelerated and the frequency enhanced by mutagens, it is presumed that genetic damage in papilloma cells plays an important role in malignant conversion. In papilloma cells lacking an activated ras^H oncogene, introduction of an exogenous ras^H oncogene leads to malignant progression. Thus, mutation and activation of this gene can contribute to early or late events in skin carcinogenesis. In either case it appears that the ras^H oncogene must cooperate with other genetic changes to contribute to the malignant phenotype.

During the last decade, chemical carcinogenesis research has substantially broadened our understanding of the cellular and molecular changes involved in cancer development and has provided new information on numerous questions in cell biology. The association of chemicals as causative factors in human cancers, the development of in vivo and in vitro experimental models, and technical advances facilitating a molecular approach to problems in cell biology have provided the impetus for progress in this research area. It is remarkable that the initial observations of the pioneers in carcinogenesis research, made more than 40 years ago, have remained valid and relevant. The newer experimental models and techniques have built on these early observations to enhance our understanding of the molecular changes that occur during cancer development. Predictably, greater insights have emphasized the finding that carcinogenesis is extraordinarily complex at the biological, cellular, and molecular levels. Yet certain generalities are becoming apparent when one compares the evolution of cancers at specific organ sites.

Lining epithelia are the major targets for cancer development in man, and both in vivo and in vitro experimental models have been established to study cancer pathogenesis in lining epithelia (Yuspa and Harris 1982). The prototype model for carcinogenesis in lining epithelia has been mouse skin (Yuspa 1986). Skin carcinogenesis has been widely studied since this target site is particularly well suited for analysis by virtue of its external location. This chapter will describe a number of aspects of the process of carcinogenesis using specific examples from the mouse skin carcinogenesis model.

The multistage development of cancer, as proposed over 40 years ago, has become commonly accepted. The linear dose-response curve for initiation of tumorigenesis, the irreversibility of the initiated state, and the persistence of initiated cells through multiple cell generations have been confirmed in many experimental models and indicate a genetic basis for initiation. In contrast, tumor promotion is reversible and requires repeated exposures to promoting agents with a defined frequency, which suggests that promotion is epigenetic. Tumor promotion has been experimentally demonstrated in mouse skin and lung, mouse and rat stomach, and rat liver, esophagus, colon, bladder, trachea, and mammary gland. These are complex epithelia in which target epithelial cells are organized in a stratifying or maturing arrangement, and frequently (but not exclusively) they undergo terminal differentiation. Such epithelia are often composed of more than one cell type or of cells in differing states of maturation and may require a tumor promoter to interrupt the cellular interactions that function to maintain tissue integrity.

In most model systems, the standard initiation and promotion protocols involving many classes of initiators and promoters primarily produce benign tumors or preneoplastic changes (Burns et al. 1983, Kaufmann et al 1985, Peraino et al. 1975). Benign tumors convert to cancers at a low frequency (1–5% of the benign tumor yield) (Scherer 1984, Taguchi et al. 1984). Most tumor promoters neither enhance the number of carcinomas that develop, even after prolonged exposure (Hennings et al. 1983, Kaufmann et al. 1985, Verma and Boutwell 1980), nor alter the preneoplastic phenotype (Goldsworthy and Pitot 1985). In contrast, the yield of malignant tumors is markedly enhanced when mice bearing benign tumors are reexposed to genotoxic initiating agents and certain genotoxic tumor promoters (such as benzoyl peroxide on mouse skin) (Hennings et al. 1983, Reiners et al. 1984, Williams et al. 1981). This implies that multiple genetic changes may be required to induce the malignant phenotype.

The potential for benign tumors to become malignant spontaneously is variable, and many benign tumors are essentially at no risk while others are at high risk (Burns et al. 1976, Hennings et al. 1985, Peraino et al. 1983, Scribner et al. 1983).

In the mouse skin model, this was determined by observing that the number of carcinomas that developed in animals receiving weak tumor promoters was identical to the number that developed in animals receiving strong promoters, although the number of benign tumors was much greater in the latter group. Thus, the benign tumors that developed in protocols with weak promoters must arise from initiated cells that are both highly sensitive to promoting agents and at high risk for malignant conversion. The determinants for these phenotypes are likely to occur at the time of initiation, perhaps as a consequence of the number of genes affected by the initiator (e.g. because of variable carcinogen delivery to individual target cells) or to the cellular function of a single genetic target of the initiator (Hennings et al. 1985, Peraino et al. 1984, Scribner et al. 1983).

THE PHENOTYPE OF INITIATION

In mouse skin, the principal benign lesions that develop as a result of initiation-promotion protocols are papillomas. The initiation of papilloma formation has an apparent one-hit dose-response pattern (Burns et al. 1983), and the tumors that form are monoclonal (Reddy and Fialkow 1983). This suggests that the papilloma represents a clonal expansion of an initiated cell. As such, the phenotype of initiation should be completely represented by the papilloma. Papillomas resemble normal epidermis in that both are composed of multiple layers of cells undergoing an orderly progression of differentiation; however in papillomas, each stratum is generally represented in greater abundance than in normal skin. Autoradiography of papillomas from animals that had received [^{3}H]thymidine shortly before sacrifice revealed that the labeling index was 10-fold higher than in normal skin. The most striking alteration, however, was the presence of thymidine-labeled cells in strata far above the basement membrane zone, a finding not observed in normal epidermis or epidermis in a nonneoplastic hyperplastic state where DNA synthesis is confined to a single layer of basal cells (Yuspa 1984). This result implies that in epidermis, initiated cells have an altered response to differentiation signals and are not obligated to cease proliferation after migration away from the basement membrane.

In cultured keratinocytes, epidermal differentiation is modulated by extracellular Ca^{2+}, and the observed changes in differentiating keratinocytes cultured in high Ca^{2+} medium (>0.1 mM Ca^{2+}) are similar to those found in vivo when normal basal cells migrate from the basement membrane. That is, in low Ca^{2+} medium (<0.1 mM Ca^{2+}) cells proliferate as basal cells and in high Ca^{2+} medium, proliferation ceases and cells terminally differentiate (Hennings et al. 1980). This seemed to be an ideal in vitro model on which to test the hypothetical link between initiation and an altered response to differentiation signals. To test the possibility that carcinogens alter the keratinocyte response to signals for terminal differentiation, basal epidermal cells were cultured in low Ca^{2+} medium, exposed to carcinogens, and then changed, stepwise, at weekly intervals into higher Ca^{2+} medium over four weeks. Carcinogen exposure in vitro resulted in the focal persistence of keratinocytes that proliferated in high Ca^{2+} medium and could be easily recognized because they stained dark red with rhodamine (Kulesz-Martin et al. 1980). A number of characteristics of this assay suggest that it selects for initiated cells: (1) cultures of basal cells isolated from initiated mouse skin and selected in high Ca^{2+} medium yield identical foci (Kawamura et al. 1985, Yuspa and Morgan 1981); (2) the number of foci increases with higher doses of carcinogen in vivo or in vitro (Kawamura et al. 1985, Kilkenny et al. 1985, Kulesz-Martin et al. 1980, 1985), (3) stronger initiators yield more foci than weaker initiators for both in vivo and in vitro exposures (Kawamura et al. 1985, Kilkenny et al. 1985), (4) for benzo[a]pyrene, the number of foci directly correlates with the extent of DNA binding after in vitro exposure (Nakayama et al. 1984), (5) the focus-forming potential of initiated skin persists for at least 10 weeks after initiation (Kawamura et al. 1985), (6) spontaneous foci develop in cultures from SENCAR mice, in which tetradecanoyl phorbol acetate (TPA) promotion induces papillomas without initiation (Kawamura et al. 1985, Yuspa and Morgan 1981), (7) foci are not tumorigenic when first formed, but cell lines derived from foci may progress to produce carcinomas upon in vivo testing (Kulesz-Martin et al. 1983). Cell lines derived from foci that show an altered response to differentiation signals and can proliferate in high Ca^{2+} medium may be considered putative initiated cells.

To compare putative initiated cells to authentic initiated cells, culture methods were developed that supported the growth of cells from papillomas induced by an initiation-promotion protocol in SENCAR mice (Yuspa et al. 1986). Six cell lines (PA, PB, PC, PD, PE and PF), which grew rapidly in low Ca^{2+} medium, were established from separate pools of papillomas. All papilloma lines responded to Ca^{2+} (>0.1 mM) as a differentiation stimulus. In the higher Ca^{2+} medium there was a 50%–95% decrease in colony-forming efficiency, a slight decrease in [^{3}H]thymidine incorporation (except for PA), and an increase in the number of cornified cells (except for early-passage PF). Epidermal transglutaminase activity, a marker for cells in an advanced stage of differentiation, increased in the presence of medium with Ca^{2+} >0.1 mM. Unlike normal cells, however, only a fraction of the cells from each of the papilloma-derived cell lines terminally differentiated in response to Ca^{2+}, while the remaining cells continued to proliferate, although at a slower rate. Thus papilloma cells and putative initiated cells have in common the ability to resist terminal differentiation induced by Ca^{2+}, but papilloma cells retain the capacity to respond partially to the Ca^{2+} signal.

Results with hematopoietic cells or adipocytes, model systems that express differentiated function in vitro, indicate that changes in the differentiation program may be an early and common change in carcinogenesis for these cell types (Sachs 1980, Scott and Maercklein 1985). However, other epithelial cells, when exposed to carcinogens in vivo or in vitro, acquired altered phenotypes of a different type, which may be recognized by selective criteria in vitro. For example, the lifespan of carcinogen-exposed tracheal epithelial cells is extended in culture, and the altered cells become less sensitive to growth factor or feeder layer requirements for clonal growth (Marchok et al. 1977, Pai et al. 1982, Thomassen et al. 1983). An altered mammary epithelial cell phenotype, resulting from limited carcinogen exposure, is manifested as a focal growth of cells with an extended lifespan in vitro, the ability of cells to form alveolar nodules in the absence of exogenous hormone in vitro, or the ability of cells to form hyperplastic nodules when transplanted to cleared mammary fat pads in vivo (Chatterjee and Banerjee 1982, Ethier 1985, Stampfer and Bartley 1985, Tonelli et al. 1979). Comparative analysis of hepatocytes from normal liver and from preneoplastic nodules indicates that the preneoplastic cells are resistant to the cytotoxic effects of certain liver carcinogens and toxins (Novicki et al. 1985). It has been proposed that resistance to cytotoxicity is associated with gamma-glutamyl transpeptidase activity, which is frequently elevated in preneoplastic mouse and rat liver foci (Hanigan and Pitot 1985). Furthermore, compared with normal liver, preneoplastic liver foci have reduced levels of enzymes required for drug metabolism (Pitot et al. 1985) and have a reduced capacity to form DNA adducts of acetylaminofluorene during continuous feeding (Huitfeldt et al. 1986). Taken together, current results in four model systems indicate that early carcinogen-induced lesions are focal, and their phenotypic character is tissue specific but generally involves an altered response to specific differentiation stimuli, altered growth requirements, or resistance to cytotoxic substances. More limited analysis suggests that similar changes occur in esophageal and lung cells from rats exposed to carcinogens in vivo (Terzaghi et al. 1981). At present, these subtle and tissue-specific changes must constitute our definition of the cellular phenotype of initiation.

THE BIOLOGY AND PHARMACOLOGY OF TUMOR PROMOTION

We have recognized agents as tumor promoters based on their capacity to increase the number or reduce the latency period of preneoplastic or neoplastic lesions after limited exposure to initiators (Table 1.1). Most promoting agents are tissue specific, do not require metabolic activation, and are commonly nonmutagenic (Diamond et al. 1980) although mutagenic agents such as ultraviolet light or bromomethylbenzanthracene may also have tumor-promoting activity (Scribner et al. 1983). Promoting agents are structurally specific so that minor changes in chemical structure markedly affect promoting activity (Diamond et al. 1980, Hecker 1978, Peraino et al. 1975). Promoters usually induce proliferation in target cells, but this effect is not sufficient for promotion (Raick 1974, Slaga et al. 1976). While the precise mechanisms of action for all promoters are not understood, the likeliest common action of these agents is to cause a selective clonal expansion of the initiated cell population resulting in a clinically evident premalignant lesion and increasing the number of cells at risk for further changes in neoplastic progression (Burns et al. 1983, Farber 1984, Moolgavkar and Knudson 1982, Yuspa et al. 1981).

Experimental data suggest that the tissue-specific action of tumor promoters may play an important role in determining the target site for tumor formation (Table 1.2). Systemic exposure to certain widely acting initiating agents produces widespread initiating mutations in rats and mice. Subsequent administration of tissue-specific promoting agents determines in which organ the tumors will develop. For example, in rats exposed to agents which can initiate both bladder and liver cells, administration of a particular bladder tumor promoter depresses the induction of liver tumors while enhancing the number of bladder tumors (Williams et al. 1983, Imaida et al. 1983). The concept that the promoting agent is a major determinant in

Table 1.1 *Experimental Promoting Agents*

Mouse Skin	*Rat Colon*
Phorbol esters	Bile acids
Anthralin	Cholestyramine
Wounding	Wounding
Benzoyl peroxide	
Cigarette smoke condensate	*Rat Bladder*
	Saccharin
Rat Liver	Cyclamate
Phenobarbital	DL-tryptophan
Dichlorodiphenyltrichloroethene (DDT)	Methyl methane sulphonate
Polychlorinated biphenyl (PCB)	
	Hormone-Dependent Tissues
Hamster or Rat Trachea	Hormones
Chronic irritation	Diet
Phorbol esters	

Table 1.2 *Promoting Agents Determine Target Site for Tumors*

Initiator	Promoter	Target Site
2-acetylaminofluorene or N-butyl-N-(4-hydroxy-butyl) nitrosamine	Phenobarbital Saccharin	Liver Bladder
Nitrosomethylurea	Phenobarbital	Liver and thyroid
Nitrosomethylurea	Saccharin	Bladder
4-acetylaminostilbene	None	Sebaceous gland
4-acetylaminostilbene	Phenobarbital	Liver
4-acetylaminostilbene	Dichlorodiphenyl-trichlorethane	Liver
4-acetylaminostilbene	Diethylstilbesterol	Liver and breast
N-nitrosodiethylamine	Phenobarbital	Liver and thyroid
N-nitrosodiethylamine	Barbital	Liver and kidney

Table 1.3 *Differential Responses of Normal and Neoplastic Cells to Tumor Promoters*

Target Tissue	Neoplastic Cell Response Compared to Normal Cell Response
Mouse and human skin (in vivo) (in vitro)	a. Resistant to promoter-induced terminal differentiation b. More resistant to promoter-mediated cytoxicity c. Enhanced sensitivity to growth stimulation by promoters
Rat liver (in vivo) (in vitro)	a. More resistant to cytotoxic agents b. Enhanced sensitivity to growth stimulation by promoters c. Altered differentiation program
Human colon (in vitro)	a. Sensitive to growth stimulation by promoter b. Stimulated to secrete proteases by promoter
Human bronchus (in vitro)	a. Resistant to promoter-induced terminal differentiation

site-specific development of cancer has important implications for human carcinogenesis.

It is unlikely that the molecular mechanism of action of promoters is common for all agents in all tissues. However, a common cellular basis for promotion is evolving from recent in vivo and in vitro experiments that have analyzed responses of carcinogen-altered (initiated), preneoplastic or benign and malignant tumor cells to promoter exposure. Normal cells from the same tissue were similarly evaluated. The data obtained from four tissues (skin, liver, colon, and bronchus) of several species indicate that during the process of carcinogenesis, altered cells become more resistant to specific or nonspecific cytocidal or cytostatic effects of certain promoters or more sensitive to the growth stimulatory effects of others (Table 1.3). These examples of differential response patterns to promoters, though specific for each agent and diverse in specific responses, would all produce the same biological effect, the selective growth of cells with the carcinogen-altered phenotype. In essence, the promoting environment in vivo would be similar to the selective growth conditions in vitro, which have been successful in elucidating the initiated phenotype. While other cellular mechanisms for tumor promotion may become obvious, current data suggest that the selective clonal expansion of the initiated cell population is the predominant action of tissue-specific tumor promoters.

The biology of phorbol ester-mediated tumor promotion in mouse skin is consistent with a process of cell selection leading to clonal expansion of initiated cells (Yuspa et al. 1981). Mouse keratinocyte cultures were used to explore the cellular basis for selection. Cultured basal cells respond heterogeneously to tumor-promoting phorbol esters (Yuspa et al. 1982). Distinct subpopulations are either induced to differentiate terminally or are stimulated to proliferate. The basis for heterogeneity in the population appears to be the maturation state of the basal cell at the time of phorbol ester exposure since (1) cells that are induced to proliferate by a single phorbol ester exposure generate new cells that can be induced to differentiate by a second exposure (Yuspa et al. 1982), and (2) advancing the maturation state of basal cells prior to phorbol ester exposure by culture in high Ca^{2+} medium leads to a uniform differentiative response at the time of promoter exposure (Yuspa et al. 1983). At the molecular level, each response appears to be mediated by distinct classes of phorbol ester receptors that also are modulated by the epidermal cell maturation state (Dunn et al. 1985).

In vivo, phorbol esters also accelerate differentiation of maturing keratinocytes (Reiners and Slaga 1983). Cells are rapidly lost from the differentiating compartment after mouse skin is exposed to phorbol esters since mRNA transcripts for differentiation-associated keratins rapidly decrease when epidermal RNA is probed with cDNA for these genes (Toftgard et al. 1985). Taken together, these results indicate that phorbol esters produce an imbalance in epidermal homeostasis because of accelerated loss of one subpopulation and selective growth of another. Our results further predict that initiated cells form a compartment that is resistant to the differentiative influences of phorbol esters.

When initiated cells and papilloma cells were examined for responses to phorbol esters by methods used to study normal cells, they were uniformly resistant to ter-

Table 1.4 *Effect of Phorbol Ester Tumor Promoters on Normal and Neoplastic Epidermal Cells*

Cell Type	Number of Individual Cell Lines Studied	% Resistant to Phorbol Ester– Induced Terminal Differentiation	% Sensitive to Phorbol Ester– Stimulated Proliferation
Normal	Multiple	0[a]	100[a]
"Initiated"	5	100	40
Papilloma-derived	7	100	85

[a] About 50% of the normal cell population terminally differentiates and the rest are mitogenically stimulated in response to phorbol esters.

minal differentiation (Table 1.4). In addition most papilloma cell lines and some initiated cell lines were sensitive to the proliferative effects of phorbol esters (Hennings et al. 1987; Yuspa et al. 1986). Furthermore, limited analysis of some of these cell lines reveals only a single class of phorbol ester receptors (Dunn et al. 1985). These results are consistent with the concept that the initiated cell compartment becomes selectively enriched with each promoter exposure to ultimately yield a benign tumor.

MALIGNANT CONVERSION AND THE NUMBER OF GENETIC CHANGES REQUIRED FOR CANCER DEVELOPMENT

Several studies have indicated that a discrete genetic change in a premalignant cell is responsible for conversion of a benign tumor to a malignant one. When animals bearing benign tumors of the skin as a result of initiation-promotion protocols are reexposed to initiating agents, they develop carcinomas with a high incidence and a short latency period (Hennings et al. 1983). Rats bearing preneoplastic foci exposed to a second initiator show neoplastic progression in the liver via an intratumoral conversion of cells in hyperplastic nodules to neoplastic cells (Scherer et al. 1984). These studies imply that two or more genetic changes are required for carcinoma formation in the liver and skin models of carcinogenesis.

Recent cell culture experiments support a two-hit model for genetic alterations in cancer development. Transfection of a single activated oncogene into primary or low-passage diploid cells produces an altered cell phenotype, but the cells are not tumorigenic (Land et al. 1983, Ruley 1983, Thomassen et al. 1985). In contrast, transfection of the same activated oncogens into premalignant (nontumorigenic) cultured cells results in their malignant (tumorigenic) conversion (Newbold and Overell 1983, Storer et al. 1986, Thomassen et al. 1985). Similarly, the cotransfection of two oncogenes into primary diploid cells is sufficient to produce the tumorigenic phenotype (Land et al. 1983, Newbold and Overell 1983, Ruley, 1983). However, the combinations of activated oncogenes required are specific, suggesting an action of each individual oncogene that complements the action of the corresponding member of the pair. If chemical carcinogens activate or otherwise mutate cellular genes to produce active oncogenes, then a two-hit theory for cancer development is supported by the transfection studies. However, the genetic damage would have to be highly selective, resulting in the activation of complementary gene pairs for the production of the cancer. Furthermore, the sequence of oncogene activation could be important in determining the final tumor phenotype.

The isolation of an activated form of the c-*ras*[H] gene from skin papillomas has provided presumptive evidence that this gene may be a target for a mutation that could constitute the initiating mutation in skin carcinogenesis (Balmain et al. 1984). Further support for this idea was provided by our studies indicating that the v-*ras*[H] gene could impart a conditional initiated phenotype on cultured keratinocytes by blocking their ability to differentiate terminally and by arresting them in a late basal cell stage of maturation (Yuspa et al. 1985). When the v-*ras*[H] gene of Harvey murine sarcoma virus (Ha-MuSV), a replication-defective transforming retrovirus, is introduced into cultured keratinocytes by a defective retroviral vector (Mann et al. 1983), skin grafts constructed with cells carrying the mutated *ras* oncogene produce papillomas on athymic mouse recipients (Roop et al. 1986). Furthermore, the exogenous oncogene appears to be regulated at the transcriptional level and is not expressed in the differentiated portions of the benign tumor, as determined by in situ hybridization studies using the v-*ras*[H] gene as a probe (Roop et al. 1986). This regulation of expression of the exogenous *ras* oncogene by the terminally differentiating tumor cells could account for the benign nature of the tumor.

While *ras* activation may be an early event in skin carcinogenesis, it is clear that not all papillomas contain an activated *ras* oncogene, and thus the benign tumor phenotype can also be achieved via other routes. When DNA from papilloma cell lines was tested in the NIH 3T3 transfection assay, active transforming activity was not detected (Harper et al. 1986). However, when the EJ *ras*[H] gene was introduced into papilloma cells by DNA transfection, transfectants showed an enhanced capacity to proliferate at clonal density under high Ca^{2+} culture conditions and formed rapidly growing, anaplastic carcinomas in nude mice. Thus, in papilloma cells, a genetic change distinct from *ras*[H] activation may produce an altered differentiation program associated with the initiation step. This genetic alteration may act in a cooperating fashion with a subsequently activated *ras* gene to result in malignant transformation. The effect of activation of the *ras* oncogene therefore varies and depends on the preexisting defined phenotype of the host cell representing specific stages in epidermal carcinogenesis. Thus, a specific temporal sequence for the activation of a particular oncogene may not be required in carcinogenesis. Mutations may occur at a single genomic locus early or late in carcinogenesis and may contribute to phenotypic progression. The phenotype which results may depend on the events that occurred previously in the target cell and on the complementary action of the specific oncogene product.

ACKNOWLEDGMENT

The studies and conclusions described in this report have resulted from experiments and discussions with a number of colleagues over several years. I am indebted to Drs. Peter Blumberg, Luigi De Luca, John Harper, Henry Hennings, Ulrike Lichti,

Douglas Lowy, Molly Kulesz-Martin, Miriam Poirier, Dennis Roop, and James Strickland for their contributions.

REFERENCES

Balmain A, Ramsden M, Bowden GT, Smith J. 1984. Activation of the mouse cellular Harvey-ras gene in chemically induced benign skin papillomas. Nature 307:658–660.

Burns F, Albert R, Altshuler B, Morris E. 1983. Approach to risk assessment for genotoxic carcinogens based on data from the mouse skin initiation-promotion model. Environ Health Perspect 50:309–320.

Burns FJ, Vanderlaan M, Sivak A, Albert RE. 1976. Regression kinetics of mouse skin papillomas. Cancer Res 36:1422–1427.

Chatterjee M, Banerjee MR. 1982. N-Nitrosodiethylamine-induced nodule-like alveolar lesion and its prevention by a retinoid in BALB/c mouse mammary glands in the whole organ in culture. Carcinogenesis 3:801–804.

Diamond L, O'Brien TG, Baird WM. 1980. Tumor promoters and the mechanism of tumor promotion. Adv Cancer Res 32:1–74.

Dunn JA, Jeng AY, Yuspa SH, Blumberg PM. 1985. Heterogeneity of [^{3}H]phorbol 12,13-dibutyrate binding in primary mouse keratinocytes at different stages of maturation. Cancer Res 45:5540–5546.

Ethier SP. 1985. Primary culture and serial passage of normal and carcinogen-treated rat mammary epithelial cells in vitro. JNCI 74:1307–1318.

Farber E. 1984. Pre-cancerous steps in carcinogenesis: their physiological adaptive nature. Biochim Biophys Acta 738:171–180.

Goldsworthy TL, Pitot HC. 1985. The quantitative analysis and stability of histochemical markers of altered hepatic foci in rat liver following initiation by diethylnitrosamine administration and promotion with phenobarbital. Carcinogenesis 6:1261–1269.

Hanigan MH, Pitot HC. 1985. Gamma-glutamyl transpeptidase—its role in hepatocarcinogenesis. Carcinogenesis 6:165–172.

Harper JR, Roop DR, Yuspa SH. 1986. Transfection of the EJ *ras*[Ha] gene into keratinocytes derived from carcinogen-induced mouse papillomas causes malignant progression. Mol Cell Biol 6:3144–3149.

Hecker E. 1978. Structure-activity relationships in diterpene esters irritant and cocarcinogenic to mouse skin. *In* Slaga TJ, Boutwell RK, eds., Carcinogenesis, A Comprehensive Survey. Raven Press, New York, pp. 11–48.

Hennings H, Michael D, Cheng C, Steinert P, Holbrook K, Yuspa SH. 1980. Calcium regulation of growth and differentiation of mouse epidermal cells in culture. Cell 19:245–254.

Hennings H, Michael D, Lichti U, Yuspa SH. 1987. Response of carcinogen-altered mouse epidermal cells to phorbol ester tumor promoters and calcium. J Invest Dermatol 88:60–65.

Hennings H, Shores R, Mitchell P, Spangler EF, Yuspa SH. 1985. Induction of papillomas with a high probability of conversion to malignancy. Carcinogenesis 6:1607–1610.

Hennings H, Shores R, Wenk M, Spangler EF, Tarone R, Yuspa SH. 1983. Malignant conversion of mouse skin tumours is increased by tumour initiators and unaffected by tumour promoters. Nature 304:67–69.

Huitfeldt HS, Spangler EF, Hunt JM, Poirier MC. 1986. Immunohistochemical localization of DNA adducts in rat liver tissue and phenotypically-altered foci during oral administration of 2-acetylaminofluorene. Carcinogenesis 7:123–129.

Imaida K, Fukushima S, Shirai T, Ohtani M, Nakanishi K, Ito N. 1983. Promoting activities of butylated hydroxyanisole and butylated hydroxytoluene on 2-stage urinary bladder carcinogenesis and inhibition of γ-glutamyl transpeptidase-positive foci development in the liver of rats. Carcinogenesis 4:895–899.

Kaufmann WK, Mackenzie SA, Kaufman DG. 1985. Quantitative relationship between hepatocytic neoplasms and islands of cellular alteration during hepatocarcinogenesis in the male F344 rat. Am J Pathol 119:171–174.

Kawamura H, Strickland JE, Yuspa SH. 1985. Association of resistance to terminal differentiation with initiation of carcinogenesis in adult mouse epidermal cells. Cancer Res 45:2748–2752.

Kilkenny AE, Morgan D, Spangler EF, Yuspa SH. 1985. Correlation of initiating potency of skin carcinogens with potency to induce resistance to terminal differentiation in cultured mouse keratinocytes. Cancer Res 45:2219–2225.

Kulesz-Martin M, Kilkenny AE, Holbrook KA, Digernes V, Yuspa SH. 1983. Properties of carcinogen altered mouse epidermal cells resistant to calcium-induced terminal differentiation. Carcinogenesis 4:1367–1377.

Kulesz-Martin M, Koehler B, Hennings H, Yuspa SH. 1980. Quantitative assay for carcinogen altered differentiation in mouse epidermal cells. Carcinogenesis 1:995–1006.

Kulesz-Martin M, Yoshida MA, Prestine L, Yuspa SH, Bertram JS. 1985. Mouse cell clones for improved quantitation of carcinogen induced altered differentiation. Carcinogenesis 6:1245–1254.

Land H, Parada LF, Weinberg RA. 1983. Tumorigenic conversion of primary embryo fibroblasts requires at least two cooperating oncogenes. Nature 304:596–602.

Mann R, Mulligan RC, Baltimore D. 1983. Construction of a retroviral packaging mutant and its use to produce helper-free defective retrovirus. Cell 33:153–159.

Marchok AC, Rhoton JC, Griesemer RA, Nettesheim P. 1977. Increased in vitro growth capacity of tracheal epithelium exposed in vivo to 7,12-dimethylbenz(a)anthracene. Cancer Res 37:1811–1821.

Moolgavkar SH, Knudson AG. 1981. Mutation and cancer: A model for human carcinogenesis. JNCI 66:1037–1052.

Nakayama J, Yuspa SH, Poirier MC. 1984. Benzo(a)pyrene-DNA adduct formation and removal in mouse epidermis in vivo and in vitro: relationship of DNA binding to initiation of skin carcinogenesis. Cancer Res 44:4087–4095.

Newbold RF, Overell RW. 1983. Fibroblast immortality is a prerequisite for transformation by EJ c-Ha-ras oncogene. Nature 304:648–651.

Novicki DL, Rosenberg MR, Michaelopoulos G. 1985. Inhibition of DNA synthesis by chemical carcinogens in cultures of initiated and normal proliferating rat hepatocytes. Cancer Res 45:337–344.

Pai SB, Steele VE, Nettesheim P. 1983. Neoplastic transformation of primary tracheal epithelial cell cultures. Carcinogenesis 4:369–374.

Peraino C, Fry RJM, Staffeldt E, Christopher JP. 1975. Comparative enhancing effects of phenobarbital, amobarbital, diphenylhydantoin, and dichlorodiphenyltrichloroethane on 2-acetylaminofluorene-induced hepatic tumorigenesis in the rat. Cancer Res 35:2884–2890.

Peraino C, Richards WL, Stevens FJ. 1983. Multistage hepatocarcinogenesis. In Slaga TJ, ed., Mechanisms of Tumor Promotion. CRC Press, Boca Raton, pp. 1–53.

Peraino C, Staffeldt EF, Carnes BA, Ludeman VA, Blomquist JA, Vesselinovitch SD. 1984. Characterization of histochemically detectable altered hepatocyte foci and their relationship to hepatic tumorigenesis in rats treated once with diethylnitrosamine or benzo(a)pyrene within one day after birth. Cancer Res 44:3340–3347.

Pitot HC, Glauert HP, Hanigan M. 1985. The significance of selected biochemical markers in the characterization of putative initiated cell populations in rodent liver. Cancer Lett 29:1–14.

Raick AN. 1974. Cell proliferation and promoting action in skin carcinogenesis. Cancer Res 34:920–926.

Reddy AL, Fialkow PJ. 1983. Papillomas induced by initiation-promotion differ from those induced by carcinogen alone. Nature 304:69–71.

Reiners JJ, Nesnow S, Slaga TJ. 1984. Murine susceptibility to two-stage skin carcinogenesis is influenced by the agent used for promotion.Carcinogenesis 5:301–307.

Reiners JJ, Slaga TJ. 1983. Effects of tumor promoters on the rate and commitment to terminal differentiation of subpopulations of murine keratinocytes. Cell 32:247–255.

Roop DR, Lowy DR, Tamborin PE, et al. 1986. An activated Harvey *ras* oncogene produces benign tumors on mouse epidermis. Nature 232:822–824.

Ruley HE. 1983. Adenovirus early region 1A enables viral and cellular transforming genes to transform primary cells in culture. Nature 304:602–606.

Sachs L. 1980. Constitutive uncoupling of pathways of gene expression that control growth and differentiation in myeloid leukemia: A model for the origin and progression of malignancy. Proc Natl Acad Sci USA 77:6152–6156.

Scherer E. 1984. Neoplastic progression in experimental hepatocarcinogenesis. Biochim Biophys Acta 738:219–236.

Scherer E, Ferigna AW, Emmelot P. 1984. Initiation-promotion-initiation. Induction of neoplastic foci within islands of precancerous liver cells in the rat. *In* Borzsonyi M, Lapis K, Day NE, Yamaski H, eds., Models, Mechanisms and Etiology of Tumor Promotion. IARC Scientific Publications, Lyon, France, pp. 57–66.

Scott RE, Maercklein PB. 1985. An initiator of carcinogenesis selectively and stably inhibits stem cell differentiation: A concept that initiation of carcinogenesis involves multiple phases. Proc Natl Acad Sci USA 82:2995–2999.

Scribner JD, Scribner NK, McKnight B, Mottet NK. 1983. Evidence for a new model of tumor progression from carcinogenesis and tumor promotion studies with 7-bromomethylbenz[a]anthracene. Cancer Res 43:2034–2041.

Slaga TJ, Scribner JD, Thompson S, Viaje A. 1976. Epidermal cell proliferation and promoting ability of phorbol esters. JNCI 57:1145–1149.

Stampfer MR, Bartley JC. 1985. Induction of transformation and continuous cell lines from normal human mammary epithelial cells after exposure to benzo[a]pyrene. Proc Natl Acad Sci USA 82:2394–2398.

Storer RC, Stein RB, Sina JF, DeLuca JG, Allen HL, Bradley MO. 1986. Malignant transformation of a preneoplastic hamster epidermal cell line by the EJ c-Ha-ras-oncogene. Cancer Res 46:1458–1464.

Taguchi T, Yokoyama M, Kitamura Y. 1984. Intraclonal conversion from papilloma to carcinoma in the skin of Pgk-1a/Pgk-1b mice treated by a complete carcinogenesis process or by an initiation-promotion regimen. Cancer Res 44:3779–3782.

Terzaghi M, Nettesheim P, Yarita T, Williams ML. 1981. Epithelial focus assay for early detection of carcinogen-altered cells in various organs of rats exposed in situ to N-nitroso-hepta-methyleneimine. JNCI 67:1057–1061.

Thomassen DG, Gilmer TM, Annab LA, Barrett JC. 1985. Evidence for multiple steps in neoplastic transformation of normal and preneoplastic Syrian hamster embryo cells following transfection with Harvey murine sarcoma virus oncogene (v-Ha-ras). Cancer Res 45:726–732.

Thomassen DG, Gray TE, Mass MJ, Barrett JC. 1983. High frequency of carcinogen-induced early, preneoplastic changes in rat tracheal epithelial cells in culture. Cancer Res 43:5956–5963.

Toftgard R, Yuspa SH, Roop DR. 1985. Keratin gene expression during mouse skin two-stage tumorigenesis. Cancer Res 45:5845:5850.

Tonelli QJ, Custer RP, Sorof S. 1979. Transformation of cultured mouse mammary glands by aromatic amines and amides and their derivatives. Cancer Res 39:1784–1792.

Verma AK, Boutwell RK. 1980. Effects of dose and duration of treatment with the tumor promoting agent, 12-0-tetradecanoyl phorbol-13-acetate on mouse skin carcinogenesis. Carcinogenesis 1:271–276.

Williams GM, Katayama S, Ohmori T. 1981. Enhancement of hepatocarcinogenesis by sequential administration of chemicals: Summation versus promotion effects. Carcinogenesis 1:1111–1117.

Williams GM, Maeura Y, Weisburger JH. 1983. Simultaneous inhibition of liver carcinogenicity and enhancement of bladder carcinogenicity of N-2-fluorenylacetamide by butylated hydroxytoluene. Cancer Lett 19:55–60.

Yuspa SH. 1984. Molecular and cellular basis for tumor promotion in mouse skin. *In* Fujiki H, Hecker E, Moore TE, Sugimura T, Weinstein IB, eds., Cellular Interactions of Environmental Tumor Promoters. Japan Science Society Press, Tokyo, pp. 315–326.

Yuspa SH. 1986. Cutaneous chemical carcinogenesis. J Am Acad Dermatol 15:1031–1044.

Yuspa SH, Harris CC. 1982. Molecular and cellular basis of chemical carcinogenesis. *In* Schottenfeld D, Fraumeni JF, eds., Cancer Epidemiology and Prevention. W. B. Saunders Co., Philadelphia, pp. 23–43.

Yuspa SH, Morgan DL. 1981. Mouse skin cells resistant to terminal differentiation associated with initiation of carcinogenesis. Nature 293:72–74.

Yuspa SH, Ben T, Hennings H. 1983. The induction of epidermal transglutaminase and terminal differentiation by tumor promoters in cultured epidermal cells. Carcinogenesis 4:1413–1418.

Yuspa SH, Ben T, Hennings H, Lichti U. 1982. Divergent responses in epidermal basal cells exposed to the tumor promoter 12-0-tetradecanoyl phorbol-13-acetate. Cancer Res 42:2344–2349.

Yuspa SH, Hennings H, Lichti U. 1981. Initiator and promoter induced specific changes in epidermal function and biological potential. J Supramol Struct Cell Biochem 17:245–257.

Yuspa SH, Kilkenny AE, Stanley J, Lichti U. 1985. Harvey and Kirsten viruses block keratinocytes in an early, phorbol ester responsive, stage of terminal differentiation. Nature 314:459–462.

Yuspa SH, Morgan D, Lichti U, et al. 1986. Cultivation and characterization of cells derived from mouse skin papillomas induced by an initiation-promotion protocol. Carcinogenesis 7:949–958.

Symposium on Fundamental Cancer Research, Vol. 39.
© 1987 by The University of Texas System Cancer Center.

2. Chromosomal Approaches to the Molecular Basis of Neoplasia

Peter C. Nowell and Carlo M. Croce

Department of Pathology and Laboratory Medicine, University of Pennsylvania and the Wistar Institute of Anatomy and Biology, Philadelphia, Pennsylvania 19104

Nonrandom patterns of chromosome abnormality in tumors are providing clues to the location of oncogenes and their activation mechanisms. Studies of translocations in Burkitt's lymphoma cells have shown that the c-*myc* proto-oncogene is consistently juxtaposed with a rearranged and transcriptionally active immunoglobulin gene locus, with resultant *myc* gene deregulation. In other B cell tumors, translocations appear to bring previously unrecognized oncogenes (*bcl*-1, *bcl*-2) into similar association with the immunoglobulin heavy-chain locus. T cell receptor genes may also "activate" known and unknown oncogenes after chromosome translocation. In chronic myelogenous leukemia, the translocated c-*abl* oncogene forms a "hybrid" gene in its new location on the Philadelphia chromosome, with altered function.

Gene amplification units, seen as cytogenetically homogeneous staining regions in chromosomes or as double-minute bodies in metaphases, can represent multiple copies of oncogenes and be important in late stages of tumor progression. Other significant alterations in gene dosage, recognized as gain or loss of all or part of a specific chromosome, also occur in human neoplasms, but their specific role in carcinogenesis is largely undefined.

Interest in the cytogenetics of tumors was reawakened in recent years as improved techniques demonstrated specific alterations in particular chromosomes that are associated, with different degrees of consistency, with specific types of tumors (Yunis 1983, Rowley 1984). These findings led to the suggestion by several workers that the nonrandom karyotypic changes might indicate sites in the genome where genes important in carcinogenesis are located, and that they might also provide clues to the mechanisms by which critical change in the function of such "oncogenes" might be mediated.

This possibility has now been explored in a number of laboratories in work focusing particularly on specific reciprocal chromosome translocations in human hematopoietic tumors such as chronic myelogenous leukemia and Burkitt's lymphoma, in which alteration in structure and/or function of proto-oncogenes, the human homologues of retroviral oncogenes, have been demonstrable. Other studies have examined chromosomal changes in tumors that involve gain or loss of genetic material, and these have suggested a critical role for oncogene dosage in the development of some neoplasms. In this brief review, we will emphasize primarily our own investigations of leukemia and lymphoma, indicating how a combined cytogenetic and molecular genetic approach can contribute to our understanding of carcinogenesis. First we will discuss our studies with human lymphomas.

BURKITT'S LYMPHOMA

About 75% of the persons with Burkitt's lymphoma in African countries in which the disease is endemic have a characteristic reciprocal translocation between chromosomes 8 and 14 in every cell of the tumor. In the remaining cases there is also a translocation involving chromosome 8, but the "donor" chromosome is either number 2 or number 22. In every instance the breakpoint in chromosome 8 is in the terminal portion of the long arm (band q24), and this is the chromosomal region to which the human homologue of the retroviral oncogene v-*myc* was mapped. At the same time, the human immunoglobulin genes were mapped to the other chromosomal regions involved in these translocations: the heavy-chain locus to band 14q32, the lambda light-chain locus to band 22q11, and kappa light-chain genes to band 2pll.

These observations suggested that an association between the c-*myc* gene and one of the immunoglobulin genes, resulting from chromosome translocation, might be significant in the pathogenesis of Burkitt's tumor, and supportive evidence has now been developed in several laboratories (Croce and Nowell 1985, Leder et al. 1983, Rabbitts et al. 1984). A combination of cytogenetic, somatic genetic, and molecular genetic techniques has been used to show that in each of these translocations a transcriptionally active and rearranged immunoglobulin gene is brought into juxtaposition with the c-*myc* gene, resulting in apparent "deregulation" of the oncogene.

In the common t(8;14) translocation, the immunoglobulin heavy-chain locus is split, and the c-*myc* oncogene, with or without major structural change, is brought into association with it (Fig. 2.1) (Rabbitts et al. 1984, Pellici et al. 1986). The circumstances are slightly different in the "variant" translocations involving chromosomes 2 and 22, but the result seems to be the same. In these instances, the kappa or lambda immunoglobulin gene is translocated to the 3' end of the c-*myc* gene, which remains on chromosome 8, often without structural alteration (Croce and Nowell 1985). Although details of these various rearrangements, and their effects, are still being investigated, it seems that in each case the c-*myc* proto-oncogene comes under the influence of enhancers in or adjacent to the immunoglobulin loci, resulting in inappropriate expression of the oncogene.

Although other factors such as chronic infection with the Epstein-Barr virus and with malaria clearly are important in the pathogenesis of Burkitt's lymphoma, particularly in Central Africa, these findings concerning the c-*myc* gene provide strong evidence for a tumorigenic effect of the chromosome translocations, and similar results in the lymphoid tumors of mice and rats support this conclusion (Klein and Klein 1985). The exact role of the *myc* gene product in the pathogenesis of Burkitt's lymphoma remains uncertain, however. The c-*myc* gene product normally functions

8   8q⁻   14   14q⁺

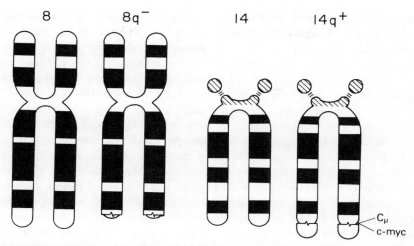

Figure 2.1. Diagram of a t(8;14) chromosome translocation in Burkitt's lymphoma, which brings the c-*myc* oncogene into juxtaposition with the immunoglobulin heavy-chain locus on chromosome 14. (From Erikson et al. 1983.)

as a nuclear protein, which seems to be important in growth regulation of lymphocytes and other cells (Kelly et al. 1983, Reed et al. 1985). Studies of the translocated c-*myc* gene on the 14q+ chromosome of Burkitt's tumor cells indicate that it can still be regulated in another cellular background (e.g., a fibroblast) but, when under the influence of an enhancing element in a B cell at the proper stage of differentiation, it does not respond to normal regulatory mechanisms (Croce and Nowell 1985). Better understanding of exactly how the deregulated oncogene, which apparently need not be structurally altered, exerts its contribution to tumorigenesis must await further clarification of the gene's normal function.

OTHER B CELL TUMORS

Because other B cell lymphomas and chronic B cell leukemias, which are more common in this country than the Burkitt's tumor, also have characteristic nonrandom translocations involving the terminal portion of the long arm of chromosome 14 (band q32), we investigated these neoplasms for possible oncogene involvement. In these tumors the donor chromosomal site, in contrast to that in the Burkitt's tumor (Yunis 1983, Rowley 1984), involves either the long arm of chromosome 11 (band q13) or the long arm of chromosome 18 (band q21). To look for significant rearrangements, the breakpoints of these translocations were molecularly cloned (Tsujimoto et al. 1985a,b), and then DNA probes flanking the breakpoints on chromosomes 11 and 18 were used to look for rearrangements of the homologous sequences in B cell lymphomas and leukemias carrying either the t(11;14) or the t(14;18) translocation. Such rearrangements were found to be clustered in short segments on chromosome 11 or chromosome 18, and the breakpoint on chromosome 14 was found consistently within the immunoglobulin heavy-chain locus.

To date, the regions of chromosomes 11 and 18 involved in these translocations have not been correlated with any known oncogenes. This may mean that they represent previously unrecognized proto-oncogenes, for which we have suggested the names bcl-1 and bcl-2, that become juxtaposed with the immunoglobulin heavy-chain locus as does the c-*myc* gene in the t(8;14) translocation of Burkitt's tumor. The bcl-2 gene has now been cloned in two other laboratories (Bakhshi et al. 1985, Cleary and Sklar 1985), and studies are under way to characterize further both of these two new putative oncogenes (Tsujimoto et al. 1985a, Cleary and Sklar 1985).

Our findings to date indicate that in both circumstances the translocation involves the J region of the immunoglobulin locus on chromosome 14. In addition, in the breakpoint regions of the translocated segments of chromosomes 11 and 18, we identified several short signal sequences typically used in V-D-J joining during normal rearrangement within the immunoglobulin heavy-chain locus during B cell differentiation. This finding indicated that the recombinase system that is normally involved in immunoglobulin gene rearrangement might erroneously use the chromosome 11 or chromosome 18 signal sequences following chromosome breakage and thus increase the probability of occurrence of the specific t(11;14) or t(14;18) translocations.

Additional progress was recently made in characterizing the bcl-2 gene. The presence of a characteristic 6-kb RNA transcript was demonstrated, with levels in leukemic cells with the t(14;18) translocation shown to be higher than in neoplastic B cells without it, which suggested deregulation of the putative oncogene. Two partially characterized protein products of the gene seem to be neither membrane nor secreted proteins. (Tsujimoto et al. 1986). These proteins apparently do not have a regulatory role within the nucleus, as does the *myc* gene product, but it may be relevant that the bcl-2 gene seems to show the same time course of expression in mitogen-stimulated normal human B cells and T cells as the c-*myc* gene (Tsujimoto et al. 1985b, and unpublished data). Even with these preliminary findings, it is clear that such molecular investigations of nonrandom chromosome translocations in human tumors promise to provide leads to genes important in human carcinogenesis that have not been identified as "oncogenes" by other approaches.

T CELL LEUKEMIAS AND LYMPHOMAS

The recent mapping of genes coding for subunits of the T cell antigen receptor provides the opportunity to ask whether oncogene "activating" mechanisms, like those described for B cell lymphomas, might also operate in T cell neoplasms. The initial findings suggest that this may be the case.

Although nonrandom chromosome changes are generally less prominent in T cell disorders, several subgroups of disorders have been described in which chromosomal translocations involve the proximal portion of the long arm of chromosome 14 (band 14q11) (Hecht et al. 1984), and the gene for the alpha chain of the T cell receptor has been mapped to this location (Croce et al. 1985). Furthermore, when we and others investigated several cases of T cell leukemia with a t(8;14) (q24;q11) translocation, we showed that this chromosomal rearrangement brings the constant portion of the alpha receptor gene into juxtaposition with the c-*myc* gene on chromosome 8, resulting in deregulation of the oncogene in a manner analogous to that of the variant translocations in Burkitt's tumor (Erikson et al. 1986a, McKeithan et al. 1986).

There seem to be other T cell neoplasms in which a nonrandom translocation involves the T-alpha locus but not a known ocogene. In certain acute T cell leukemias of childhood, for example, a t(11;14) (p13;q11) translocation was shown to interrupt the alpha locus of the T cell receptor, but no gene has been assigned to the involved region of the short arm of chromosome 11 (Erikson et al. 1985, Lewis et al. 1985). We also have similar data from a patient with acute lymphocytic leukemia and a t(14;20) (q11;q13) rearrangement (Erikson et al. 1986b). Although still very preliminary, these findings suggest that the alpha T cell receptor gene may have the same "activating" role in T cell neoplasms as do the immunoglobulin genes in B cell tumors, and that this approach may lead to the identification of new oncogenes specific for T cell disorders.

Two other genes for T cell receptor subunits were recently mapped as well, the beta locus to the long arm of chromosome 7 (band q35) and the gamma locus to the short arm of the same chromosome (7p13) (Isobe et al. 1985, Morton et al. 1985). A few T cell tumors have been described in which these chromosome regions are involved in translocations (Sanger et al. 1986), and it seems likely that a role similar to that of the alpha locus will be demonstrated in these cases.

The investigations are complicated by the fact that all three sites of T cell receptor genes, as well as the chromosome 14q32 region, appear to be unusually fragile in the T cells of normal individuals as well as in individuals with such chromosome fragility syndromes as ataxia telangiectasia. Metaphases with rearrangements involving these four sites are therefore observed with greater than random frequency in cultures of mitogen-stimulated *non*neoplastic lymphocytes. This may simply reflect the effect of the physiologic recombination that occurs normally at these sites during lymphocyte differentiation, but such rearrangements are also observed in T cell neoplasms.

In the latter circumstance, it is not yet clear exactly what genes are involved or their contribution to leukemogenesis. For example, inversion of a portion of chromosome 14, bringing the 14q11 region into juxtaposition with the 14q32 region, is relatively common in chronic T cell neoplasms (Isobe et al. 1985, Morton et al. 1985). In one case studied in detail (Baer et al. 1985, and unpublished data), this rearrangement was shown to bring T-alpha sequences into the immunoglobulin heavy-chain locus, but it is not clear how such an association might confer a selective growth advantage on the involved cell, and whether the same relationship exists in other cases with an inverted chromosome 14.

There may be other critical genes in the 14q32 region (Croce et al. 1985). We observed a similar circumstance in a patient with B cell chronic lymphocytic leukemia in which a t(14;22) translocation brought lambda light-chain sequences into the heavy-chain locus (Nowell et al. 1986, and unpublished data), but apparently this is a rare phenomenon in B cell tumors. The next several years should provide considerable additional interesting information on the molecular genetics of both B cell and T cell neoplasms.

MYELOID LEUKEMIA

A variety of nonrandom translocations have been associated with subgroups of acute nonlymphocytic leukemia. In several instances, preliminary attempts were made to demonstrate specific oncogene involvement along with alteration in gene function, but so far no clear relationship has been confirmed. One suggestion, for example, is that the c-*erb*A oncogene and other genes in the same chromosome region might be significantly involved in the t(15;17) (q22;q21) translocation characteristic of acute promyelocytic leukemia (Dayton et al. 1984, Coussens et al. 1985, Huebner et al. 1986). Other associations have been postulated for the t(8;21) (q22;q22) translocation in acute myelocytic leukemia and the inverted chromosome 16 in acute myelomonocytic leukemia (Rowley 1984, Le Beau et al. 1985). By the time this brief review appears, specific information concerning one or more of these chromosome translocations and the involved oncogenes may be forthcoming.

Such information is already available with respect to chronic myelogenous leukemia (CML), which is marked by the characteristic t(9;22) (q34;q11) translocation that produces the Philadelphia (Ph) chromosome in nearly every typical case (Yunis 1983, Rowley 1980). The chromosomal breakpoints in this rearrangement have been mapped, and the results indicate that the c-*abl* proto-oncogene is regularly translocated from its normal location on chromosome 9 (band q34) to a very restricted region of chromosome 22 that has been termed the "breakpoint cluster region" or bcr (Groffen et al. 1984).

This joining region on chromosome 22 has now been cloned and a novel 8-kb mRNA containing both bcr and *abl* sequences demonstrated (Shtivelman et al. 1985). This "hybrid" transcript codes for a protein of increased molecular weight, with markedly elevated tyrosine kinase activity as compared to the normal c-*abl* gene product. These findings in CML thus demonstrate a tumorigenic chromosomal translocation in which both structure and function of the oncogene product are modified, compared with the Burkitt's tumor translocations in which the *myc* gene product appears substantially unaltered.

We and others are extending these studies to other neoplasms with translocations involving the same band of chromosome 22 (q11), including cases of acute *lymphocytic* leukemia in which a Ph chromosome is present, the variant cases of Burkitt's lymphoma discussed above, and Ewing's sarcoma (Croce and Nowell 1985, Erikson et al. 1986b, Emanuel et al. 1986). Our findings and those of others indicate that, although the chromosome breakpoints and even the translocations involving chromosome 22 in different tumors may appear microscopically identical, they are heterogeneous at the molecular level. For example, we have data on five cases of acute lymphocytic leukemia (ALL) in which a characteristic t(9;22) (q34;q11) translocation, producing a typical Ph chromosome, demonstrates such heterogeneity (Erikson et al. 1986b). In two adult patients, the molecular data indicated that the translocation was identical to that in CML, involving the bcr, but in two children and one young adult the breakpoint in 22q was shown to be proximal to the bcr. The breakpoint in chromosome band 22q11 in these Ph-positive ALL cases also seemed to be distal to that of the t(8;22) (q24;q11) translocation in the variant Burkitt's lymphomas in which the lambda immunoglobulin light-chain locus is involved (Croce and Nowell 1985, Cannizzaro et al. 1985). Interestingly, the t(11;22) (q23;q11) translocation that characterizes Ewing's sarcoma and certain neuroepitheliomas also seems, at the molecular level, to involve a different breakpoint in band 22q11, but this is *distal* to the bcr (Emanuel et al. 1986). These observations serve to emphasize the fact that chromosomal translocations may help to identify sites of oncogene involvement in carcinogenic rearrangements, but that detailed molecular characterization is required for confirmation and clarification.

GENE DOSAGE AND CHROMOSOMAL ABNORMALITIES

Reciprocal translocations are not the only cytogenetic alterations identified as occurring nonrandomly in neoplasia and presumably resulting in significant alteration of oncogene function (Sandberg 1980). Other abnormalities include chromosomal trisomies and monosomies representing gain or loss of a whole chromosome, as well as gains or deletions of a chromosome portion. In any of these circumstances, the oncogenic effect is assumed to result from gain or loss of a single copy of one or more oncogenes, but there is of course the possibility of significant, concurrent structural genetic alterations. There is also a group of chromosomal aberrations, the gene amplification units, in which one can cytogenetically recognize a major change in gene dosage. These units appear in neoplastic metaphases as homogeneous staining regions (HSR) or abnormal banding regions (ABR) on chromosomes, or as multiple small, paired bodies known as double minutes (DM). Earlier studies of such structures in established cell lines indicated that they may be relatively labile and indeed seem to be alternative forms of amplification of the same gene within a cell population (Balaban-Malenbaum and Gilbert 1977, Kaufman et al. 1979, Biedler et al. 1983). These structures do not show the same consistent localization within the genome as do other cytogenetic rearrangements that contribute to carcinogenesis, but they have been shown, in some cases, to involve human proto-oncogenes. For example, in certain neuroblastomas, amplification of c-*myc* has been demonstrated, as well as a homologous gene, now called N-*myc,* located on chromosome 2 (Schwab et al. 1983). Similar data have been reported for other solid tumors (Alitalo et al. 1983, Little et al. 1983), such as small cell lung carcinoma, and occasionally in leukemic cell lines as well. We observed amplified c-*myc* as an HSR on chromosome 8 in the HL-60 cell line derived from a patient with acute promyelocytic leukemia (Nowell et al. 1983) and amplification of the translocated c-*abl* oncogene as an ABR in cells derived from a patient with Ph-positive CML (Selden et al. 1983).

Such gene amplification units seem more characteristically associated with the more aggressive stages of clinical disease, indicating their role in the clinical and biological progression of neoplasia (Seeger et al. 1985). Based on the limited information available the suggestion is that, among the various mechanisms for altering oncogene function, chromosome translocation may be particularly relevant in early tumor development and gene amplification in later phases.

Relatively little is known concerning the genes involved in those nonrandom cytogenetic alterations that appear to involve the gain or loss of a single gene copy, even though some of these are among the most frequent nonrandom karyotypic alterations in human neoplasia. Trisomy 8, for example, is the most common cytogenetic change in human acute leukemia, and it also occurs in a variety of other tumors (Yunis 1983, Sandberg 1980). Trisomy 12 is the most common abnormality in the B cell form of chronic lymphocytic leukemia (Nowell et al. 1986, Juliusson et al. 1985), and trisomy 7 is frequently observed in the advanced stages of malignant melanoma (Becher et al. 1983, Balaban et al. 1986). In a collaborative study of the latter tumor, we observed that this extra dosage of chromosome 7 was consistently associated with expression on the melanoma cells of the receptor for epidermal growth factor (EGF) (Koprowski et al. 1985). Because the human proto-oncogene c-erbB is located on the short arm of chromosome 7 and appears to code for a portion of the EGF receptor (Downward et al. 1984), this may be the first example of a single extra copy of an oncogene resulting in significantly altered function and contributing to additional selective growth advantage for already malignant cells. As noted above, however, it is not yet clear whether one or more of the EGF receptor gene copies represented in these melanomas also has a structural change.

The same considerations apply to certain tumors in which a whole chromosome or a chromosomal segment is lost. This phenomenon has been observed in some human leukemias and preleukemias, as well as in such solid malignancies as Wilms' tumor and retinoblastoma. A number of research groups are currently investigating both inherited and sporadic cases of retinoblastoma, and it seems that a necessary step in the tumorigenic process is gene deletion or mutation in the proximal portion of the long arm of both number 13 chromosomes, at band q14 (Yunis and Ransey 1978). These lesions may be visible to the cytogeneticists or may be submicroscopic. The suggestion is that loss or inactivation of negative regulatory genes through such deletions may foster tumor development by derepressing other critical genes (Knudson 1985, Atkin 1985). Attempts are under way to characterize the specific genes involved in the pathogenesis of retinoblastoma, as well as in such similar circumstances as the preleukemic "5q— syndrome," which may involve deletion of genes that regulate myeloid proliferation and differentiation (Neinhuis et al. 1985, Huebner et al. 1985).

DISCUSSION

During the past several years, information on the karyotypic characteristics of mammalian tumors has contributed significantly to the recognition and investigation of individual genes important in carcinogenesis (Klein and Klein 1985, Bishop 1985, Weinberg 1985). Such "oncogenes" were first identified in mammalian cells through their homology with retroviral oncogenes and through their capacity for cellular transformation in transfection assays, but cytogenetic findings are now helping to indicate the location in the human genome of previously unrecognized proto-oncogenes (Croce and Nowell 1985, Klein and Klein 1985, Bishop 1985), as well as indicating the involvement of some of the previously known oncogenes in human tumorigenesis. In addition, these chromosome studies expand our understanding of the various mechanisms by which a significant change in the function of a proto-oncogene can be brought about within the potentially neoplastic cell. Certain of these "activating" processes are obviously not visible at the chromosome level, such as point mutation and promoter insertion. Cytogenetic investigations have provided evidence, however, on the importance of other mechanisms, such as alteration in gene dosage (through amplification, trisomy, or deletion), as well as of reciprocal chromosomal translocation with or without structural change in the oncogene (Croce and Nowell 1985, Klein and Klein 1985, Seeger et al. 1985).

As we said earlier, the most extensive work to date in correlating the cytogenetic and molecular findings in chromosome translocations has been done in certain lymphomas and chronic myelogenous leukemia. These data showed that this type of somatic genetic rearrangement represents an important mechanism whereby oncogene function can be critically altered and made to contribute to the development of human malignancies. The findings in these neoplasms also demonstrated different mechanisms of "activation" of a proto-oncogene following chromosome transloca-tion. In Burkitt's lymphoma, the c-*myc* oncogene appears to be deregulated by its juxtaposition to a rearranged and transcriptionally active immunoglobulin gene, without necessarily requiring significant structural change in the proto-oncogene for this effect (Croce and Nowell 1985). In chronic myelogenous leukemia, in contrast, the "hybrid" gene produced as a result of the translocation event yields an altered c-*abl* oncogene product with a resultant change in function (Shtivelman et al. 1985). Until more information is available on the molecular genetics of other nonrandom translocations in human tumors, it is not possible to generalize as to the relative frequency of different effects of such rearrangements.

It is somewhat ironic that, as investigators interested in the mechanisms of carcino-genesis can for the first time approach identification of the specific genes and gene products involved in the process, new layers of complexity are uncovered. The new information is not making the problem simpler. We must continue to recognize the multiple steps and factors involved in cellular transformation and subsequent tumor development. These involve not only genetic alterations in the tumor cells, but they also reflect changes in growth regulatory mechanisms of the host (Klein and Klein 1985, Nowell 1986). We continue to have large gaps in knowing the sequence of events in normal growth regulation, and although the products of a number of onco-genes have been identified as nuclear proteins, tyrosine kinases, growth factors, or their receptors (Klein and Klein 1985, Bishop 1985, Ford and Maizel 1985), it is not yet clear exactly how their alteration results in abnormal growth patterns. Ulti-mately, from the combined approaches of multiple disciplines, including tumor cytogenetics, certain patterns will emerge, and clinical applications may follow. Until then, many exciting areas are open for exploration, and premature generaliza-tion should be avoided.

SUMMARY

Karotypic studies of various tumors have revealed nonrandom patterns of chromosome abnormality. These are providing clues to the location of genes important in carcinogenesis (oncogenes) and to mechanisms for their activation. Translocations within the chromosomal complement have been particularly revealing. Molecular investigations of the translocations in Burkitt's lymphoma cells have shown, for example, that the c-*myc* proto-oncogene is consistently brought into juxtaposition with a rearranged and transcriptionally active immunoglobulin gene locus, with resultant deregulation of the *myc* gene. A similar phenomenon probably occurs in a number of other B cell tumors, with translocations involving the immunoglobulin heavy-chain locus and previously unrecognized oncogenes (e.g., *bcl*-1, *bcl*-2). Recent data from T cell tumors suggest that T cell receptor genes, and particularly the T alpha gene, may similarly "activate" both known and unknown oncogenes following chromosome translocation. In nonlymphocytic leukemias, the tumorigenic effect of translocations may be mediated by different mechanisms. In chronic myelogenous leukemia, for example, the translocated c-*abl* oncogene forms a "hybrid" gene in its new location, with altered function. Molecular data on other nonlymphocytic leukemias are incomplete.

Among the somatic genetic alterations important in carcinogenesis, translocations are not the only ones recognizable as karyotypic changes. Gene amplification units, seen as homogeneous staining regions in chromosomes or as double minute bodies in metaphases, have been demonstrated to represent multiple copies of oncogenes, particularly in such solid tumors as neuroblastoma and small cell lung cancer. These amplification units seem most commonly associated with late stages of tumor progression. Other alterations in gene dosage, recognized as gain or loss of all or part of a specific chromosome, also occur nonrandomly in human leukemias and other neoplasms, and they indicate a selective growth advantage for cells carrying these changes. To date, however, the specific genes and mechanisms involved have not been defined. Investigation of tumor chromosomes helps to pinpoint human oncogenes, and detailed study of their carcinogenic role must then be pursued with molecular techniques.

REFERENCES

Alitalo A, Schwab M, Lin CC, Varmus HE, Bishop JM. 1983. Homogeneously staining chromosomal regions contain amplified copies of an abundantly expressed cellular oncogene (c-myc) in malignant neuroendocrine cells from a human colon carcinoma. Proc Natl Acad Sci USA 80:1707–1711.

Atkin NB. 1985. Antioncogenes. Lancet II:1189–1190.

Baer R, Chen K-C, Smith SD, Rabbitts TH. 1985. Fusion of an immunoglobulin variable gene and a T cell receptor constant gene in the chromosome 14 inversion associated with T cell tumors. Cell 43:705–713.

Bakhshi A, Jensen JP, Goldman P, Wright JJ, McBride OW, Epstein AL, Korsmeyer SJ. 1985. Cloning the chromosomal breakpoint of t(14;18) human lymphomas:clustering J_H on chromosome 14 and near a transcriptional unit on 18. Cell 41:899–906.

Balaban G, Herlyn M, Clark WH, Nowell PC. 1986. Karyotypic evolution in human malignant melanoma. Cancer Genet Cytogenet 19:113–122.

Balaban-Malenbaum G, Gilbert F. 1977. Double minute chromosomes and the homogeneously staining regions in chromosomes of a human neuroblastoma cell line. Science 198:739–741.

Becher R, Gibas Z, Karakousis C, Sandberg AA. 1983. Nonrandom chromosome changes in malignant melanoma. Cancer Res 43:5010–5016.

Biedler JL, Malera PW, Spengler BA. 1983. Chromosome abnormalities and gene amplification: comparison of antifolate-resistant and human neuroblastoma cell systems. In Rowley JD, Ultmann JB, eds., Chromosomes and Cancer: From Molecules to Man. Academic Press, New York, pp. 117–138.

Bishop JM. 1985. Trends in oncogenes. Trends in Genetics 1:245–249.

Cannizzaro LA, Nowell PC, Belasco JB, Croce CM, Emanuel BS. 1985. The breakpoint in 22q11 in a case of Ph-positive acute lymphocytic leukemia interrupts the immunoglobulin light chain gene cluster. Cancer Genet Cytogenet 18:173–177.

Cleary ML, Sklar J. 1985. Nucleotide sequence of a t(14;18) chromosomal breakpoint in follicular lymphoma and demonstration of a breakpoint cluster region near a transcriptionally active locus on chromosome 18. Proc Natl Acad Sci USA 82:7439–7443.

Coussens L, Yang-Feng TL, Lioao Y-C, Chen E, Gray A, McGrath J, Seeburg PH, Libermann TA, Schessinger J, Francke U, Levinson A, Ullrich A. 1985. Tyrosine kinase receptor with extensive homology to EGF receptor shares chromosomal location with neu oncogene. Science 230:1132–1139.

Croce CM, Nowell PC. 1985. Molecular basis of human B cell neoplasia. Blood 65:1–7.

Croce CM, Isobe M, Palumbo A, Puck J, Ming J, Tweardy D, Erikson J, Davis M, Rovera G. 1985. Gene for alpha-chain of human T-cell receptor: location on chromosome 14 region involved in T-cell neoplasms. Science 227:1044–1047.

Dayton AI, Selden JR, Laws G, Dorney DJ, Finan J, Tripputi P, Emanuel BS, Rovera G, Nowell PC, Croce CM. 1984. A human c-erbA oncogene homologue is closely proximal to the chromosome 17 breakpoint in acute promyelocytic leukemia. Proc Natl Acad Sci USA 81:4495–4499.

Downward J, Yarden Y, Mayes E, Scrace G, Totty N, Stockwell P, Ullrich A, Schlessinger J, Waterfield MD. 1984. Close similarity of epidermal growth factor receptor and v-erbB oncogene protein sequences. Nature 307:521–527.

Emanuel BS, Nowell PC, Croce CM, Israel MI. 1986. Translocation breakpoint mapping: molecular and cytogenetic studies of chromosome 22. Cancer Genet Cytogenet 19:81–92.

Erikson J, ar-Rushdi A, Drwinga H. Nowell P, Croce C. 1983. Transcriptional activation of the translocated c-myc oncogene in Burkitt lymphoma. Proc Natl Acad Sci USA 80: 820–824.

Erikson J, Williams DL, Finan J, Nowell PC, Croce CM. 1985. Locus of the alpha-chain of the T-cell receptor is split by chromosome translocation in T-cell leukemias. Science 229:784–786.

Erikson J, Finger L, Sun L, ar-Rushdi A, Nishikura K, Minowada J, Finan J, Emanuel BS, Nowell PC, Croce CM. 1986a. C-myc deregulation by translocation of the alpha locus of T cell receptor in T cell leukemias. Science 232:884–886.

Erikson J, Griffin CG, ar-Rushdi A, Valtieri M, Hoxie J, Finan J, Emanuel BS, Rovera G, Nowell PC, Croce CM. 1986b. Heterogeneity of chromosome 22 breakpoint in Ph-positive acute lymphocytic leukemia. Proc Natl Acad Sci USA 83:1807–1811.

Ford R, Maizel A, eds. 1985. Mediators in Cell Growth and Differentiation. Raven Press, New York.

Groffen J, Stephenson JR, Heistercamp N, DeKlein A, Barton CR, Grosveld G. 1984. Philadelphia chromosomal breakpoints are clustered within a limited region, bcr, on chromosome 22. Cell 36:93–99.

Hecht F, Morgan R, Hecht BK-M, Smith SD. 1984. Common region on chromosome 14 in T-cell leukemia and lymphoma. Science 226:1445–1446.

Huebner K, Isobe M, Croce CM, Golde DW, Kaufman SE, Gasson JC. 1985. The human gene encoding GM-CSF is at 5q21-q32, the chromosome region deleted in the 5q− anomaly. Science 230:1282–1285.

Huebner K, Isobe M, Chao M, Bothwell M, Ross AH, Finan J, Hoxie JA, Sehgal A, Buck CR, Lanahan A, Nowell PC, Koprowski H, Croce CM. 1986. The nerve growth factor receptor gene is at human chromosome region 17q12-17q22, distal to the chromosome 17 breakpoint in acute leukemias. Proc Natl Acad Sci USA 83:1403–1407.

Isobe M, Emanuel BS, Erikson J, Nowell PC, Croce CM. 1985. Location of gene for beta subunit of human T cell receptor at band 7q35, a region prone to rearrangements in T cells. Science 228:580–582.

Juliusson G, Robert K-H, Ost A, Friberg K, Biberfeld P, Nilsson B, Zech L, Gahrton G. 1985. Prognostic information from cytogenetic analysis in chronic B-lymphocytic leukemia and leukemic immunocytoma. Blood 65:134–141.

Kaufman RJ, Brown PC, Schimke RT. 1979. Amplified dihydrofolate reductase genes in unstably methotrexate-resistant cells are associated with double minute chromosomes. Proc Natl Acad Sci USA 76:5669–5673.

Kelly K, Cochran BH, Stiles CD, Leder P. 1983. Cell-specific regulation of the c-myc gene by lymphocyte mitogens and platelet-derived growth factor. Cell 35:603–610.

Klein G, Klein E. 1985. Evolution of tumors and the impact of molecular oncology. Nature 315:190–195.

Knudson AG. 1985. Hereditary cancer, oncogenes, and antioncogenes. Cancer Res 45:1437–1443.

Koprowski H, Herlyn M, Balaban G, Parmiter A, Ross A, Nowell PC. 1985. Expression of the receptor for epidermal growth factor correlates with increased dosage of chromosome 7 in malignant melanoma. Somatic Cell Molec Genet 11:297–302.

Le Beau MM, Diaz MO, Karin M, Rowley JD. 1985. Metallothionein gene cluster is split by chromosome 16 rearrangements in myelomonocytic leukaemia. Nature 313:709–711.

Leder P, Battey J, Lenoir G, Moulding C, Murphy W, Potter H, Stewart T, Taub R. 1983. Translocations among antibody genes in human cancer. Science 222:765–771.

Lewis WH, Michalopoulos EE, Williams DL, Minden MD, Mak TW. 1985. Breakpoints in the human T-cell antigen receptor alpha-chain locus in two T-cell leukaemia patients with chromosomal translocations. Nature 317:544–546.

Little CD, Nau NM, Carney DN, Gazdar AF, Minna JD. 1983. Amplification and expression of the c-myc oncogene in human lung cancer cell lines. Nature 306:194–196.

McKeithan TW, Shima EA, Le Beau MM, Minowada J, Rowley JD, Diaz MO. 1986. Molecular cloning of the breakpoint junction of a human chromosomal 8;14 translocation involving the T-cell receptor alpha-chain gene and sequences on the 3′ side of MYC. Proc Natl Acad Sci USA 83:6636–6640.

Morton CC, Duby AD, Eddy RL, Shows TB, Seidman JG. 1985. Genes for the beta chain of human T-cell antigen receptor map to regions of chromosomal rearrangement in T cells. Science 228:582–585.

Neinhuis AW, Bunn HF, Turner PH, Gopal TV, Nash WG, O'Brien SJ, Sherr CJ. 1985. Expression of the human c-fms proto-oncogene in hematopoietic cells and its deletion in the 5q− syndrome. Cell 42:421–428.

Nowell PC. 1986. Mechanisms of tumor progression. Cancer Res 46:2203–2207.

Nowell P, Finan J, Dalla-Favera R, Gallo R, ar-Rushdi A, Ramanczuk P, Selden J, Emanuel B, Rovera G, Croce C. 1983. Association of amplified oncogene c-myc with an abnormally banded chromosome 8 in a human leukemia cell line. Nature 306:494–497.

Nowell PC, Vonderheid EC, Besa E, Hoxie J, Moreau L, Finan J. 1986. The most common chromosome change in 86 chronic B-cell or T-cell tumors: a 14q32 translocation. Cancer Genet Cytogenet 19:219–227.

Pelicci P-G, Knowles DM, Magrath I, Dalla-Favera R. 1986. Chromosomal breakpoints and structural alterations of the c-*myc* locus differ in endemic and sporadic forms of Burkitt lymphoma. Proc Natl Acad Sci USA 83:2984–2988.

Rabbitts TH, Foster A, Hamlyn P, Baer R. 1984. Effect of somatic mutation within translocated c-myc genes in Burkitt's lymphoma. Nature 309:592–597.

Reed JC, Nowell PC, Hoover RG. 1985. Regulation of c-myc mRNA levels in normal human lymphocytes by modulators of cell proliferation. Proc Natl Acad Sci USA 82:4221–4224.

Rowley JD. 1980. Ph-positive leukaemia, including chronic myelogenous leukaemia. Clin Haematol 9:55–86.

Rowley JD. 1984. Biological implications of consistent chromosome rearrangements in leukemia and lymphoma. Cancer Res 44:3159–3168.

Sandberg AA. 1980. The Chromosomes in Human Cancer and Leukemia. Elsevier, New York.

Sanger WG, Weisenburger DD, Armitage JO, Purtilo DT. 1986. Cytogenetic abnormalities in noncutaneous peripheral T-cell lymphoma. Cancer Genet Cytogenet 23:53–59.

Schwab M, Alitalo K, Klempnauer K-H, Varmus HE, Bishop JM, Gilbert F, Brodeur G, Goldstein M, Trent J. 1983. Amplified DNA with limited homology to myc cellular oncogene is shared by neuroblastoma cell lines and a neuroblastoma tumor. Nature 305:245–248.

Seeger RC, Brodeur GM, Sather H, Dalton A, Siegel SE, Wong KY, Hammond D. 1985. Association of multiple copies of the N-*myc* oncogene with rapid progression of neuroblastomas. N Engl J Med 313:1111–1116.

Selden J, Emanuel B, Wang E, Cannizzaro L, Palumbo A, Erikson J, Nowell P, Rovera G, Croce C. 1983. Amplified C-lambda and c-*abl* genes on the same marker chromosome in K562 leukemic cells. Proc Natl Acad Sci USA 80:7289–7292.

Shtivelman E, Lifshitz B, Gale RP, Cananni E. 1985. Fused transcript of *abl* and *bcr* genes in chronic myelogenous leukaemia. Nature 315:550–554.

Tsujimoto Y, Jaffe E, Cossman J, Gorham J, Nowell PC, Croce CM. 1985a. Clustering of breakpoints on chromosome 11 in human B cell neoplasms with the t(11;14) chromosome translocation. Nature 315:340–343.

Tsujimoto Y, Cossman J, Jaffe E, Croce CM. 1985b. Involvement of the *bcl*-2 gene in human follicular lymphoma. Science 228:1440–1443.

Tsujimoto Y, Croce CM. 1986. Analysis of the structure, transcripts, and protein products of *bcl*-2, the gene involved in human follicular lymphoma. Proc Natl Acad Sci USA 83:5214–5218.

Weinberg RA. 1985. The action of oncogenes in the cytoplasm and nucleus. Science 230:770–783.

Yunis JJ. 1983. The chromosomal basis of human neoplasia. Science 221:227–236.

Yunis J, Ransey N. 1978. Retinoblastoma and subband deletion of chromosome 13. Am J Dis Child 132:161–163.

Symposium on Fundamental Cancer Research, Vol. 39.
© 1987 by The University of Texas System Cancer Center.

3. Critical Genetic Determinants and Molecular Events in Multistage Skin Carcinogenesis

Thomas J. Slaga, John O'Connell, Joel Rotstein, George Patskan, Rebecca Morris, Claudio M. Aldaz, and Claudio J. Conti

*The University of Texas System Cancer Center,
Science Park—Research Division, Smithville, Texas 78957*

Carcinogenesis can be operationally and mechanistically divided into at least three major stages—initiation, promotion, and progression. Variations among stocks and strains of mice to susceptibility to multistage skin and liver carcinogenesis appear to be more related to alterations in tumor promotion than tumor initiation; however, the critical events have not been determined. In the mouse skin model the first stage is thought to involve the interaction of a tumor initiator with the genetic material of stem cells leading to an alteration in some aspect of growth control, differentiation, or both. The major effect of tumor promoters, regardless of the type, is the specific expansion of the initiated stem cells in the skin. This appears to occur by both direct and indirect mechanisms that involve the loss of glucocorticoid receptors, differentiation alterations, a direct growth stimulation of the initiated cells, or selective cytotoxicity. The progression stage is characterized by a high level of genetic instability that produces a number of chromsomal alterations. These changes may be responsible for the loss of the high-molecular-weight keratin proteins and filaggrin, increase in gamma-glutamyl-transpeptidase activity, and changes in oncogene expression in squamous cell carcinomas. We have found that a high percentage of squamous cell carcinomas have a trisomy in chromosome 2 that carries both *src* and *abl* genes and an increased expression of *src* and *abl*. We have also found increased Ha-*ras* on RNA expression in both papillomas and squamous cell carcinomas. We suggest that the genetic instability of the initiated cells is responsible for most observed changes during skin carcinogenesis.

Chemical carcinogenesis in several different tissues in a number of species is a multistage process that can be divided into three major stages: initiation, promotion, and progression. An important aspect of this multistage process is the suggestion that both genetic and epigenetic mechanisms are important in carcinogenesis. Altered growth control and differentiation leading to a more embryonic phenotype appear to be critical consequences of the genetic and epigenetic changes.

Skin tumors can be induced by the sequential application of a subthreshold dose of a carcinogen (initiation stage) followed by repetitive treatment with a noncarcinogenic promoter (promotion stage). The initiation phase requires only a single application of either a direct or an indirect carcinogen and is essentially an irreversible step; the promotion phase, however, is initially reversible but later becomes irreversible. A single large dose of a carcinogen such as 7,12-dimethylbenz(a)anthrancene (DMBA) is capable of inducing skin tumors in mice, in which papillomas occur after a relatively short latency period (10–20 weeks). Carcinomas develop after a longer period (20–60 weeks). If this dose is lowered it becomes necessary to administer DMBA repeatedly in order to induce tumors. If it is progressively reduced, a subthreshold dose of DMBA is reached that will not give rise to tumors over the lifespan of the mouse. If either croton oil or a phorbol ester, such as 12-0-tetradecanoylphorbol-13-acetate (TPA), is then applied repeatedly to the backs of mice previously initiated with a single subthreshold dose of DMBA, multiple papillomas appear after a short latency period, followed by squamous cell carcinomas after a much longer period. If the promoter is repeatedly applied but there is no initiation by DMBA, there are generally no tumors or only a few, but they never exhibit a dose-response relationship (Slaga et al. 1981, 1982). If the mice are initiated with a subthreshold dose of a carcinogen, such as DMBA, there is an excellent dose response using TPA as the promoter (Slaga et al. 1982). Likewise, there is a very good dose response with benzo(a)pyrene [B(a)P] or DMBA, as a tumor initiator, when the promoter dose is held constant (Slaga et al. 1982).

The order of treatments of the initiator and promoter is also important. If repetitive applications of the promoter are adminstered before initiation, no tumors will develop. The real hallmark of the two-stage carcinogenesis system in mouse skin relates to the irreversibility of tumor initiation. A delay of up to one year between the application of the initiator and the beginning of the promoter treatment provides a tumor response similar to that observed when the promoter is given only one week following initiation (Slaga et al. 1982). Unlike the initiation phase, the promotion stage is reversible and requires a certain frequency of application in order to induce tumors (Slaga et al. 1982). In this chapter, the progression stage is defined as those events occurring after the initial appearance of a skin tumor and represents the transition from a benign (papilloma) to malignant (squamous cell carcinoma) lesion and finally to metastatic tumors.

CRITICAL TARGETS AND EVENTS IN SKIN TUMOR INITIATION

The tumor initiation stage in mouse skin seems to be an irreversible stage that probably involves a somatic mutation in some aspect of epidermal growth control or epidermal differentiation (Slaga et al. 1982). Extensive data have revealed a good correlation between the carcinogenicity of many chemical carcinogens and their mutagenic activities (Slaga et al. 1982). Most tumor initiating agents either generate or are metabolically converted to electrophilic reactants, which bind covalently to cellular DNA and other macromolecules (Miller and Miller 1976). Previous studies have demonstrated a good correlation between the skin tumor initiating activities of several polycyclic aromatic hydrocarbons (PAH) and their abilities to bind covalently to DNA (Slaga et al. 1982).

Dark Cells as Targets of Tumor Initiation

We have recently found that skin tumor initiation probably occurs in dark basal keratinocytes, since a good correlation exists between the degree of tumor initiation and the number of dark basal keratinocytes present in the skin (Slaga and Klein-Szanto 1983). The dark basal keratinocytes are present in the skin in large numbers during embryogenesis, in moderate numbers in newborns, in low numbers in young adults, and in very low numbers in older adults, a finding which suggests that these cells may be epidermal stem cells (Klein-Szanto and Slaga 1981, Slaga and Klein-Szanto 1983). The initiating potential of mouse skin decreases with the age of the mouse, to the point that it is very difficult to initiate tumors in mice older than one year. At that time, dark basal keratinocytes are extremely rare.

In a series of experiments, Goerttler and coworkers (1976), performed transplacental initiation of fetal epidermis with low doses of DMBA at different days of gestation. The sensitivity to initiation that was demonstrated postnatally by TPA topical treatments varied markedly according to the prenatal day of initiation. Our recent results with SENCAR mice (Slaga and Klein-Szanto 1983) are similar to those reported by Goerttler. In addition, we found that the pattern of sensitivity to initiation was extremely similar to the pattern of dark cell distribution reported by Klein-Szanto and Slaga (1981)—gradual increases from day 12 of gestation, maximum number at day 19 of gestation, and sudden drop thereafter. Van Duuren et al. (1975), using a two-stage carcinogenesis protocol (DMBA plus TPA), showed that age at promotion plays a critical role in tumor production. A general decrease in tumor incidence occurred with increasing age at the time promotion was observed. These coincidences point to the fact that dark cells, being less-differentiated keratinocytes, are more susceptible to the action of carcinogens and promoters; therefore, the number of dark cells available at initiation or promotion or both could be a critical factor for efficient tumor induction. In this context it is interesting to note that although carcinogenic doses of DMBA induce a large number of dark cells, initiating doses (subcarcinogenic doses) do not alter the percentage of dark basal cells in the epidermis. These data suggest that the number of dark basal cells, "stem cells," correlates with the degree of tumor initiation.

Carcinogen-Retaining Epidermal Cells

There is substantial evidence that suggests that normal basal keratinocytes within epidermal proliferative units and hair follicles form a maturation series of slowly cycling, self-renewing stem cells, proliferative but nonrenewing transit (amplifying) cells, and postmitotic maturing keratinocytes in mice (Christophers 1971, Mackenzie 1970, Marks 1976). Although previous studies have demonstrated the fairly uniform initial binding of radioactively labeled carcinogens throughout the epidermal basal layer (Hamilton and Potten 1972, Potten 1975), very little is known about possible relationships between keratinocyte maturity and the persistence of radioactively labeled carcinogen. Therefore, we have used ^{3}H- and ^{14}C-labeled B(a)P to identify in the dorsal epidermis of mouse cells retaining labeled carcinogen (Morris et al. 1986). The distribution and persistence of radioactively labeled B(a)P in the skin of adult SENCAR female mice were investigated by autoradiography of epidermal whole mounts and cross-sections at intervals following a single initiating application of B(a)P. One day after treatment, the entire thickness of the skin was labeled; the grain density was greatest over hair follicles, sebaceous glands, and interfollicular epidermis. At one and two weeks, decreases in the nuclear grain density were consistent with the overall pattern of epidermal renewal. One month after treatment, carcinogen label-retaining cells made up approximately 2% of the interfollicular basal cells. They were also present in the hair follicles; approximately 4% and 5% of basal cells in the infundibulum and external root sheath, respectively. They were rare in the germ region and dermal papilla. Carcinogen label-retaining cells were compared with slowly cycling [^{3}H]thymidine-retaining cells and "maturing" basal cells, two distinct proliferative subsets of adult murine epidermis. Carcinogen label-retaining cells were found to have characteristics of the slowly cycling cells. First, most of the carcinogen-labeled nuclei were found in the central regions of the epidermal proliferative units, and second treatment of the carcinogen label-retaining cells with 2 μg of TPA elicited labeled mitoses within one day and a general decrease in grain density over basal nuclei. In contrast, four days after a single injection of [^{3}H]thymidine "maturing" basal cells were found at the periphery of the epidermal proliferative units. Within one day after treatment with 2 μg of TPA, "maturing" basal cells were displaced to the suprabasal layers. Double isotope-double emulsion autoradiographs demonstrated doubly labeled cells one month after continuous labeling with [^{3}H]thymidine and [^{14}C]B(a)P. They provide evidence that the radioactive carcinogen is retained by the slowly cycling [^{3}H]thymidine-retaining cells. These observations suggest that a slowly cycling population of epidermal cells may be relevant to the initiation phase of two-stage carcinogenesis (Morris et al. 1986).

CRITICAL EVENTS IN SKIN TUMOR PROMOTION

Biochemical and Morphologic Events

Extensive data suggest that skin tumor promoters do not bind *covalently* to DNA and are not mutagenic but rather bring about a number of important epigenetic changes (Slaga et al. 1982). In addition to causing inflammation and epidermal hyperplasia, phorbol ester and other tumor promoters produce many other morphological and biochemical changes in the skin. Of the observed promoter-related effects on the skin—the induction of epidermal cell proliferation, ornithine decarboxylase (ODC), and subsequent polyamines—prostaglandins and dark basal keratinocytes have the best correlation with promoting activity (Slaga et al. 1981, 1982). In addition to the induction of dark cells, which are normally present in large numbers in embryonic skin, many other embryonic conditions appear in adult skin after treatment with tumor promoters and may be a consequence of the alteration in differentiation.

It is difficult to determine which of the many effects associated with tumor promotion are, in fact, essential components of the promotion process. A good correlation appears to exist between promotion and epidermal hyperplasia (Slaga et al. 1981). However, some agents that induce epidermal cell proliferation do not promote carcinogenesis (Slaga et al. 1982). Nevertheless, it should be emphasized that all known skin tumor promoters do induce epidermal hyperplasia (Slaga et al. 1981). O'Brien et al. (1975) have reported an excellent correlation between the tumor-promoting ability of various compounds and their ability to induce ODC activity in mouse skin. However, mezerein, a diterpene similar to TPA but with weak promoting activity, induced ODC to levels that were comparable to those induced by TPA (Mufson et al. 1979). Raick (1974) found that phorbol ester tumor promoters induced the appearance of "dark basal cells" in the epidermis, whereas ethylphenylpropiolate (EPP), a nonpromoting epidermal hyperplastic agent, did not. Wounding induced a few dark cells, which seemed to correlate with its ability to be a weak promoter (Raick 1974). In addition, a large number of these dark cells are found in papillomas and carcinomas (Slaga et al. 1982). Klein-Szanto et al. (1980) reported that TPA induced about three to five times the number of dark cells as mezerein, which was the first major difference found between these compounds.

A number of other important epigenetic changes in the skin, such as membrane and differentiation alterations and increases in protease activity, cAMP-independent protein kinase activity, and phospholipid synthesis, have been caused by promoters (Slaga et al. 1982). In addition, the skin tumor promoters cause a decrease in epidermal superoxide dismutase and catalase activities, as well as a decrease in the number of glucocorticoid receptors and a decreased response of G_1 chalone in adult skin (Slaga 1983). The phorbol ester tumor promoters and teleocidin-induced changes seem to be mediated by their interaction with specific membrane receptors, whereas many of the other promoters, such as benzoyl peroxide and anthralin, do not act through this receptor, but may involve a free radical mechanism (Slaga 1983).

Studies using cell culture systems have suggested that the primary action of tumor-promoting phorbol esters takes place at the cell surface (Slaga 1983). The exposure of a variety of cell culture systems to phorbol ester tumor promoters brings about an increased membrane fluidity, increased uptake of 2-deoxyglucose and ^{32}Pi and ^{86}RB$^+$, inhibition of epidermal growth factor (EGF) binding to cellular receptors, synergistic interaction with growth factors, altered cell adhesion and uncoupling of B-adrenergic receptors, an increased turnover of membrane phospholipids, and increased prostaglandin synthesis (Slaga 1983). In general, there exists a good correlation between the tumor-promoting activity of phorbol esters on mouse skin and their effects on membrane structure and function.

Specific Receptors

Specific receptors with a high affinity for phorbol esters have been demonstrated not only in mouse skin but also in crude membrane fractions or intact cells from a variety of cultured cells and tissues (Blumberg 1981). A close association between the binding sites of phorbol esters, calcium, and phospholipid-dependent protein kinase (C kinase) has also been found. This protein kinase is activated by unsaturated diacylglycerol, which may be transiently formed during the receptor-mediated turnover of phosphatidylinositol (Blumberg 1981). Castagna et al. (1982) have shown that TPA can directly activate this protein kinase in vitro in the absence of diacylglycerol. Subsequently, Niedel et al. (1983) and Ashendel et al. (1983) have reported the copurification of phorbol ester receptors with protein kinase C. These results suggest that protein kinase C is the phorbol ester receptor. Because of the importance of protein kinase C in normal growth control, its activation could be a critical event in all carcinogenesis.

Cell-to-Cell Communication

A number of studies showing that tumor promoters inhibit cell-to-cell communication provide an important clue to the process of tumor promotion, since cell-to-cell communication is thought to play a crucial role in the control of cell proliferation and differentiation (Loewenstein 1981). The observation that TPA and other tumor promoters inhibit metabolic cooperation between cells in culture has recently provided evidence for this important event (Troska et al. 1982). Tumor promoters also reversibly inhibit both the formation and maintenance of electrical coupling of cultured human epithelial cells (Enomoto et al. 1981). A block in intercellular communication may enhance tumor formation in the skin by producing, for example, a disturbance in proliferation and cell differentiation. Consistent with this hypothesis is the finding that TPA seems to induce the appearance of intercellular spaces between epidermal cells of mouse skin and impairs epidermal cell differentiation (Slaga 1983).

Differentiation

Several investigations have revealed that altered differentiation plays a critical role in tumor promotion and carcinogenesis in general. Tumor promoters transiently induce in epidermal and other cells a set of phenotypic changes that resemble those found in embryonic and in malignant cells. Raick (1974) found that tumor-promoting agents induced in basal keratinocytes certain morphologic changes resembling those found in embryonic, papillomas, and carcinoma cells. Klein-Szanto et al. (1980) found that tumor promoters increased the number of dark basal keratinocytes in adult skin, which were normally in high numbers in embryonic skin, papillomas, and carcinomas. Theoretically, modulation of the commitment of differentiation or differentiation potential of subpopulations of keratinocytes could result in the accumulation of subpopulations of initiated cells. Reiners and Slaga (1983) found that tumor promoters commit a subpopulation of basal cells to terminal differentiation and accelerate the rate of differentiation of committed cells. Yuspa et al. (1982) also found that tumor promoters induced subpopulations of basal cells in culture to differentiate. This could happen through an important mechanism in the expansion of the initiated cell population. In this regard, Yuspa and Morgan (1981) found that initiated epidermal cells in culture do not differentiate under a physiological stimulus to differentiate (e.g., high calcium).

Table 3.1 *Mechanisms of Selection of Initiated Epidermal Stem Cell by Skin Tumor Promoters*

1. Some tumor promoters may have a direct effect on initiated stem cells (dark cells?) causing them to divide and increase in number.
2. Tumor promoters convert some basal keratinocytes to an embryonic phenotype similar to the dark cells and thereby supply a positive environment for the initiated dark cells to increase in number.
3. Tumor promoters stimulate terminal differentiation of some epidermal cells and thus decrease a feedback mechanism to cell proliferation.
4. Some tumor promoters have a selective cytotoxic effect that may cause initiated cells to increase in number.

Genetic Effects

Recent reports suggest that tumor promoters may also have an effect on the genetic material of cells. Free radicals may be the cause of the many genetic effects. Some promoters, such as benzoyl peroxide, spontaneously give rise to free radicals, whereas others, such as phorbol ester and teleocidin-type promoters, may give rise to free radicals because of their clastogenic effect (Cerutti et al. 1983). Oxidized lipids and oxygen radicals, induced by the clastogenic effect of TPA, could have a direct effect on the genetic material. Tumor promoters have caused gene amplification (Varshavsky 1981), mitotic aneuploidy in yeast (Parry et al. 1981), synergistic interactions with viruses in enhancing cell transformation (Fischer and Weinstein 1979), enhancement of irreversible anchorage–independent growth in mouse epidermal cell lines (Colburn et al. 1979), and sister chromatid exchange (Kinsella and Radman 1978).

The epigenetic effects of the tumor promoters are reversible and thus may be more important in the earlier stages of promotion, since promotion itself is reversible for a reasonable period of time. On the other hand, the genetic effects of the tumor promoters may be responsible for the irreversible portion or late state of promotion.

Overall, the critical aspect of skin tumor promotion and possibly tumor promotion in other systems is the selective expansion of the initiated cells by the tumor promoter. Table 3.1 summarizes various possible mechanisms of selection of initiated cells.

CRITICAL EVENTS IN SKIN TUMOR PROGRESSION

Although many studies have been directed toward understanding the mechanisms involved in skin tumor initiation and promotion, only a few have been performed on the progression stage of skin carcinogenesis. Table 3.2 summarizes some of the important characteristics of skin papillomas and carcinomas in order to emphasize the events that seem to be critical in the conversion from papilloma to carcinoma. There are several events that occur during tumor promotion that continue or are even exaggerated during tumor progression. These events include an increase in dark cells, a loss of glucocorticoid receptors, and an increase in polyamines and prostaglandins (Slaga 1983).

Table 3.2 *Characteristics of Skin Tumors*

Benign Papillomas

1. Papillomas have a large number of dark cells.
2. There is a loss of glucocorticoid receptors.
3. There is a high level of polyamines and prostaglandins.
4. Approximately 80% of the papillomas induced by the two-stage protocol have high-molecular-weight keratins and filaggrin and do not have GGT; 20% have reverse conditions.
5. Approximately 50% of papillomas induced by the two-stage protocol express Ha-*ras* RNA.
6. Some papillomas are reversible.
7. Treatment of papillomas with MNNG, ENU, benzoyl peroxide, and H_2O_2 increases the conversion of papillomas to carcinomas.
8. Early papillomas (10 weeks) are well differentiated hyperplastic lesions during promotion with mild or no cellular atypia, whereas late ones (40 weeks) are dysplastic, show atypia, and are aneuploid.

Carcinomas

1. Carcinomas have a large number of dark cells.
2. They all lack glucocorticoid receptors.
3. There are high levels of polyamines and prostaglandins.
4. They all lack high-molecular-weight keratins and filaggrin.
5. They all contain GGT.
6. Approximately 67% of carcinomas induced by two-stage protocol express Ha-*ras* RNA. Complete carcinogenesis protocol by MNNG does not increase the expression of Ha-*ras* RNA but does increase the expression of *src* and *abl*.
7. MNNG treatment of mice with carcinomas increases their metastatic potential.
8. They all are aneuploid with some nonrandom chromosomal changes, such as trisomy in chromosomes 2 and 6.

There are also a number of changes that occur very late in the carcinogenesis process that are related to the conversion of benign tumors to malignant tumors. We have found that all squamous cell carcinomas lack several differentiation product proteins, such as high-molecular-weight keratins (60,000–62,000) and filaggrin, but have gamma glutamyltransferase (GGT). However, only about 20% of the papillomas generated by an initiation-promotion protocol exhibit a similar condition (Klein-Szanto et al. 1983, Nelson et al. 1982). Before visible tumors are observed using the initiation-promotion protocol, these conditions seem to be normal, suggesting that these changes are very late responses (Nelson et al. 1982).

Balmain and coworkers (1984) found that a percentage of papillomas and carcinomas induced by DMBA-TPA contained elevated levels of Ha-*ras* transcripts, when compared with normal epidermis. Furthermore, the tumor DNA was capable of malignantly transforming NIH 3T3 cells in DNA transfection studies (Balmain and Pragnell 1983). Studies in our laboratory (Pelling et al. 1984) indicate that initiation alone or repetitive TPA treatments are insufficient to turn on the expression of the Ha-*ras* oncogene in adult SENCAR mouse epidermis. Initiation followed by either one or six weeks of TPA treatment also failed to activate Ha-*ras* expression. Like Balmain, we observed elevated levels of Ha-*ras* RNA in a percentage of papillomas and carcinomas tested. We also found that the expression of c-*src* and c-*abl* are increased in the majority of carcinomas examined (Patskan et al. 1985). It still remains to be determined, however, if oncogene activation plays a critical role in multistage skin carcinogenesis.

Hennings and coworkers (1983) reported that if mice with papillomas are treated repetitively with N-methyl-N-nitrosoquanidine (MNNG), a significant increase in the conversion of papillomas to carcinomas occurs. We have also found similar results with limited treatment of MNNG, as well as with ethylnitrosourea (ENU) and benzoyl peroxide and with hydrogen peroxide (O'Connell et al. 1986a, b). This type of treatment (initiation-promotion-initiation) produces a carcinoma response similar to complete carcinogenesis, i.e., the repetitive application of a carcinogen, such as DMBA or MNNG, probably supplies continuous initiating and promoting influences. The reason that a different type of promoter, like benzoyl peroxide, or a nonpromoter, like hydrogen peroxide, can increase the conversion of papillomas to carcinomas is currently unknown.

The mechanisms involved in tumor progression in the mouse skin system are unclear. The carcinogens ENU and MNNG and the peroxides are all genotoxic compounds. Chromosomal studies have shown that squamous cell carcinomas are highly aneuploid lesions often exhibiting hyperdiploid stem cell lines (Aldaz et al. 1987). Although early papillomas (10 weeks of promotion) are diploid, they progressively show chromosomal changes and eventually all become aneuploid after 30 to 40 weeks of promotion (Aldaz et al. 1987). Additional evidence does indicate that specific chromosome alterations, trisomy of chromosomes 2 and 6, may be markers of malignancy, since they are present in a high percentage of squamous cell carcinomas (Conti et al. 1986). Whether the genotoxic effects of the agents used in progression experiments are able to induce such specific alterations is unknown.

In addition to chromosomal alterations, squamous cell carcinomas exhibit a number of changes in protein expression, including the lack of high-molecular-weight keratins (Klein-Szanto 1984) and filaggrin (Mamrack et al. 1984), and the presense of GGT. Possibly these phenotypic changes are the result of the gene alterations and rearrangements and can be induced by genotoxic agents. When ENU and benzoyl were used as "progressors" to induce keratoacanthomas, histologic and cytochemical studies showed a high percentage of GGT-positive tumors. This may reflect a novel expression of this enzyme in benign lesions (O'Connell et al. 1986a).

A different mechanism of genetic alteration that could be relevant to progression is change in the methylation state of DNA. Preliminary evidence from this laboratory has indicated that a gradient in DNA methylation exists from normal mouse epidermis to papillomas to carcinomas; carcinomas are highly undermethylated (La Peyre JN, unpublished data). Both of the "progressors," ENU and MNNG used in this study inhibited methylation by blocking DNA methyltransferase activity (Wilson and Jones 1983).

Another hypothesis for the action of "progressor" agents is related to their high degree of cytotoxicity. In this model for progression, many highly cytotoxic agents selectively or nonselectively kill cells within a tumor, allowing the growth of more malignant cells, or they kill normal cells, reducing the constraints against expansion along the border between normal and tumor tissue. Both alternatives assume that cells capable of invasion preexist within the benign tumor or that expansion of tumor clones increases the chance of the natural progression of cells toward malignancy. We are currently testing a number of cytotoxic agents for activity during the progression stage.

GENETIC DETERMINANTS OF SKIN CARCINOGENESIS

There is a fairly good correlation in any given species between the amount of carcinogen bound to DNA and the tumor response of the carcinogen (Miller and Miller 1976). Furthermore, for any individual stock or strain of mouse, it has been generally observed that there is an excellent correlation between the amount of polycyclic aromatic hydrocarbons (PAH) bound to DNA and the skin tumor response (Slaga et al. 1982). However, this correlation between DNA binding and tumor response breaks down when a comparison is made between mouse strains or stocks that differ in their tumor response to two-stage or to complete carcinogenesis (Slaga et al. 1982). Phillips et al. (1978) have demonstrated that the kinetics of binding of DMBA to the DNAs of C57BL/6, DBA/2, and Swiss mice were virtually identical in terms of formation and removal of adducts with time (Table 3.3). The kinetics of DMBA binding to epidermal DNA and removal in SENCAR and CD-1 mice are also similar to the above strains of mice (Slaga et al. 1982). Although these data are far from conclusive, they suggest that some aspects of initiation are probably similar in strains and stocks of mice that differ in their response to two-stage or complete carcinogenesis. Drinkwater and Ginsler (1984) also reported that the kinetics of N,N-diethylnitrosourea (DEN) binding to liver DNA in two different strains of mice were very similar even though their susceptibility to DEN carcinogenicity was quite different. When newborn male C57BL/6 and C3H mice were injected with DEN, the mean liver tumor multiplicities at 32 weeks of age were 0.33 and 35 tumors/animal, respectively (Drinkwater and Ginsler 1984). This suggests that the difference in susceptibility to DEN is related to an event or events after initiation.

Importance of Tumor Promotion in Inter- and Intraspecies Differences

Most of the data that suggest the importance of tumor promotion in the inter- and intraspecies differences in carcinogenesis come from studies using skin as the target tissue. Furthermore, most of the data on two-stage skin carcinogenesis are based

Table 3.3 *The Binding of 7,12-Dimethylbenz(a)anthracene to the DNA of the Skin of Mice of Different Strains*

Strain	DMBA Bound (pmol/mg DNA) in Mouse Skin			
	Hours			
	12	24	96	192
C57BL	22.0	52.4	19.2	8.3
DBA/2	30.5	41.0	19.0	10.5
Swiss	21.5	40.2	18.2	9.8

Adapted from Phillips et al. 1978.

on using a PAH as the initiator and croton oil or a phorbol ester as the promoter (Slaga and Fischer 1983). Under these conditions mice are much more sensitive than hamsters and rats (Slaga and Fischer 1983). It is possible that if a different initiator or promoter were used, the sensitivity to two-stage carcinogenesis in various species could be quite different.

DiGiovanni and coworkers (1984) have examined the sensitivity of SENCAR, DBA/2, and C57BL/6 mice to skin tumor promotion by TPA. Their results, as well as others (DiGiovanni et al. 1984, Reiners et al. 1983), have shown that SENCAR mice are more sensitive to TPA promotion than DBA/2 mice if DMBA is used as the initiator. However, DiGiovanni and coworkers (1984) have also found that the DBA/2 mice are as sensitive to TPA promotion as SENCAR mice if a direct-acting carcinogen such as MNNG is used as the initiator. When either of these initiators were used, the C57BL/6 mice were resistant to TPA promotion (DiGiovanni et al. 1984). In addition, these investigators found that susceptibility to TPA promotion seems to be inherited as an autosomal semidominant trait in crosses between C57BL/6 and DBA/2 mice. Furthermore, susceptibility to liver tumor induction in various mouse strains and hybrids also seems to be related to tumor promotion (Drinkwater and Ginsler 1984).

SENCAR mice are sensitive to complete carcinogenesis as well as to two-stage carcinogenesis (Slaga and Fischer 1983). C57BL/6 mice are also very resistant to two-stage skin carcinogenesis by B(a)P-TPA. Even high initiating doses of BP (1600 moles) and high promoting doses of TPA (10 μg) are ineffective in causing skin tumors. However, C57BL/6 mice do respond to complete carcinogenesis by B(a)P (Reiners et al. 1984). This unequal susceptibility to complete and two-stage carcinogenesis within a stock or strain of mice strongly suggests that promotional stages of complete and two-stage carcinogenesis are dissimilar. In addition, differences in sensitivity to initiation and promotion between mice may be due to alterations in the promotional stage of two-stage carcinogenesis. In this regard, we have recently found that benzoyl peroxide is an effective promoter in C57BL/6 and SENCAR mice when using DMBA as the initiator. In the DMBA-benzoyl peroxide experiments, SENCAR and C57BL/6 mice have similar tumor responses (Reiners et al. 1984).

In order to understand the difference in susceptibility to TPA promotion in SENCAR and C57BL/6 mice, Slaga and coworkers (1983) examined a number of biochemical and morphologic responses assumed to be markers for skin tumor promotion. After a single topical treatment with TPA to SENCAR and C57BL/6 mice, however, there were some differences in hyperplasia, dark cells, and ornithine decarboxylase activity; the differences were not great enough to account for the difference in tumor response (Slaga and Fischer 1983). Furthermore, C57BL/6 mice contain specific receptors for TPA (Slaga and Fischer 1983, Blumberg 1981). The reason TPA is not an effective promoter in C57BL/6 mice may be related to its lack of ability to induce sustained hyperplasia after repetitive TPA treatment (Slaga and Fischer 1983). Likewise, Sisskin et al. (1982) showed that the hamster, a species that is resistant to two-stage carcinogenesis, responds to a single treatment of TPA but loses its responsiveness to repetitive treatment.

An inbred strain of SENCAR mice was developed that is much more sensitive to two-stage skin carcinogenesis protocols than the outbred parental stock (Fischer et al. 1987). These mice, SSIN, are at least three times more sensitive than outbred SENCAR. Furthermore, there is a much greater increase in ODC and hyperplasia as a result of promotion by TPA in SSIN than in outbred SENCAR. These data also suggest that the susceptibility to skin carcinogenesis is related to tumor promotion.

ACKNOWLEDGMENT

The research was supported by Public Service grants CA-34890, CA-34962, and CA-34521 from the National Cancer Institute. We gratefully acknowledge our past and present technicians, students, postdoctoral fellows, and collaborators who contributed to these studies. We also thank Christie Hoy and Karen Engel for their help in preparing and typing this manuscript.

REFERENCES

Aldaz CM, Conti CJ, Klein-Szanto AJP, Slaga TJ. 1987. Progressive dysplasia and aneuploidy are hallmarks of mouse skin papillomas: Relevance to malignancy, Proc Natl Acad Sci USA 84:2029–2032.

Ashendel CL, Staller JM, and Boutwell RK. 1983. Solubilization, purification, and reconstitution of a phorbol ester receptor from the particulate protein fraction of mouse brain. Cancer Res 43:4227–4332.

Balmain A, Pragnell ID. 1983. Mouse skin carcinomas induced *in vivo* by chemical carcinogens have a transforming Harvey-*ras* oncogene. Nature 303:72–74.

Balmain A, Ramsden M, Bowden GT, Smith J. 1984. Activation of the mouse cellular Harvey-ras gene in chemically induced benign skin papillomas. Nature 307:658–660.

Blumberg PM. 1981. *In vitro* studies on the mode of action of the phorbol esters, potent tumor promoters. CRC Crit Rev Toxicol 9:153–197.

Castagna M, Takai Y, Kaibuchi K, Sano K, Kikkawa U, Nishizuka Y. 1982. Direct activation of calcium-activated phospholipid-dependent protein kinase by tumor promoting phorbol esters. J Biol Chem 257:7847–7851.

Cerutti P, Emerit I, Amstad P. 1983. Membrane-mediated chromosomal damage. *In* Weinstein IB, Vogel H, eds., Genes and Proteins in Oncogenesis. Proceedings of P & S Biomedical Sciences Symposium. Academic Press, New York, pp. 55–67.

Christophers E. 1971. Cellular architecture of the stratum corneum. J Invest Dermatol 56:165–170.

Colburn NH, Former BF, Nelson KA, Yuspa SH. 1979. Tumor promoter induces anchorage independent irreversibily. Nature 266:589–591.

Conti CJ, Aldaz CM, O'Connell J, Klein-Szanto AJP, Slaga TJ. 1986. Aneuploidy, an early event in mouse skin tumor development. Carcinogenesis 7:1845–1848.

DiGiovanni J, Prichett WP, Decina PC, Diamond, PL. 1984. DBA/2 mice are as sensitive as SENCAR mice to skin tumor promotion by 12-0-tetradecanoylphorbol-13-acetate. Carcinogenesis 5:1493–1498.

Drinkwater N, Ginsler J. 1984. Genetic control of susceptibility to liver tumor induction in mice (Abstract). Proceedings of the American Association for Cancer Research 25:126.

Enomoto T, Sasaki Y, Shiba Y, Kanno Y, Yamasaki H. 1981. Tumor promoters cause a rapid and reversible inhibition of the formation and maintenance of electrical cell coupling in culture. Proc Natl Acad Sci USA 78:5628–5632.

Fischer SM, O'Connell JF, Conti CJ, et al. 1987. Characterization of an inbred strain of the SENCAR mouse that is highly sensitive to phorbol esters. Carcinogenesis (in press).

Fischer PB, Weinstein IB. 1979. Chemical viral interactions and multistep aspects of cell transformation. *In* Montesano H, Bartsh H, Tomates L, eds., Molecular and Cellular Aspects of Carcinogen Screening Tests. IARC Scientific Publications, Lyon, pp. 113–131.

Goerttler K, Loehrke H. 1976. Diaplacental carcinogenesis: initiation with the carcinogens dimethylbenzanthracene (DMBA) and urethane during fetal life and postnatal promotion with the phorbol ester TPA in a modified 2 stage Berenblum-Mottram experiment. Virchows Arch[A] 372:29–38.

Hamilton E, Potten CS. 1972. Influence of hair plucking on the turnover time of the epidermal basal layer. Cell Tissue Kinet 5:505–517.

Hennings H, Shores R, Wenk ML, Spangler EF, Tarone R, Yuspa SH. 1983. Malignant conversion of mouse skin tumours is increased by tumour initiators and unaffected by tumour promoters. Nature 304:67–69.

Kinsella AR, Radman M. 1978. Tumor promoter induces sister chromatid exchanges: Relevance to mechanisms of carcinogenesis. Proc Natl Acad Sci USA 75:6149–6153.

Klein-Szanto AJP. 1984. Morphological evaluation of tumor promoter effects on mammalian skin. *In* Slaga TJ, ed., Mechanisms of Tumor Promotion, vol. II. CRC Press, Boca Raton, p. 418.

Klein-Szanto AJP, Slaga TJ. 1981. Numerical variation of dark cells in normal and chemically induced hyperplastic epidermis with age of animal and efficiency of tumor promoter. Cancer Res 41:4437–4440.

Klein-Szanto AJP, Major SM, Slaga TJ. 1980. Induction of dark keratinocytes by 12-0-tetradecanoylphorbol-13-acetate and mezerein as an indicator of tumor promoting efficiency. Carcinogenesis 1:399–406.

Klein-Szanto AJP, Nelson RG, Shah Y, Slaga TJ. 1983. Keratin modifications and GGT activity as indication of tumor progression in skin papillomas. JNCI 70:161–168.

Loewenstein WR. 1981. Junctional intercellular communication: The cell-to-cell membrane channel. Physiol Rev 61:829–913.

Mackenzie IC. 1970. Relationship between mitosis and the structure of the stratum corneum in mouse epidermis. Nature 226:653–655.

Mamrack MD, Klein-Szanto AJP, Reiners JJ Jr, Slaga TJ. 1984. Alteration in the distribution of the epidermal protein filaggrin during two stage chemical carcinogenesis in the SENCAR mouse skin. Cancer Res 44:2634.

Marks F. 1976. Epidermal growth control mechanisms, hyperplasia, and tumor promotion in the skin. Cancer Res 36:2636–2643.

Miller EC, Miller JA. 1976. The metabolism of chemical carcinogens to reactive electrophiles and their possible mechanism of action in carcinogenesis. *In* Searle CE, ed., Chemical Carcinogens. ACS, Washington, pp. 737–762.

Morris RJ, Fischer SM, Slaga TJ. 1986. Evidence that a slowly cycling subpopulation of adult murine epidermal cells retains carcinogen. Cancer Res 46:3061–3066.

Mufson RA, Fischer SM, Verma AK, Gleason GL, Slaga TJ, Boutwell RK. 1979. Effects of 12-0-tetradecanoylphorbol-13-acetate and mezerein on epidermal ornithine decarboxylase activity, isoproterenol-stimulated levels of cyclic adenosine 3:5-monophosphate, and induction of mouse skin tumors. Cancer Res 39:4791–4795.

Nelson KG, Stephenson KB, Slaga TJ. 1982. Protein modification induced in mouse epidermis by potent and weak tumor-promoting hyperplasiogenic agents. Cancer Res 42:4164–4174.

Niedel JE, Kuhn LJ, Vandenback GR. 1983. Phorbol diester receptor copurifies with protein kinase C. Proc Natl Acad Sci USA 80:36–40.

O'Brien TG, Simsiman RC, Boutwell RK. 1975. Induction of the polyamine biosynthetic enzymes in mouse epidermis by tumor promoting agents. Cancer Res 35:1662–1670.

O'Connell JF, Klein-Szanto AJP, DiGiovanni DM, Fries JW, Slaga TJ. 1986a. Malignant progression of mouse skin papillomas treated with ethylnitrosourea, N-methy-N′-nitrosoguanidine or 12-0-tetradecanoylphorbol-13-acetate. Cancer Lett 30:269.

O'Connell JF, Klein-Szanto AJP, DiGiovanni DM, Fries JW, Slaga TJ. 1986b. Enhanced malignant progression of mouse skin tumors by the free-radical generator benzoyl peroxide. Cancer Res 46:2863.

Parry JM, Parry EM, Barrett JC. 1981. Tumor promoters induce mitotic aneuploidy in yeast. Nature 294:263–265.

Patskan GJ, Pelling JC, Nairn RS, Slaga TJ. 1985. Altered oncogene expression in mouse skin squamous cell carcinomas. Presented at the Pennsylvania State University Fourth Summer Symposium in Molecular Biology, State College, PA.

Pelling JC, Hixson DC, Nairn RS, Slaga TJ. 1984. Altered gene expression during two-stage tumorigenesis in SENCAR mouse skin (Abstract). Proceedings of the American Association of Cancer Research 25:78.

Phillips DH, Grover PL, Sims P. 1978. The covalent binding of polycyclic hydrocarbons to DNA in the skin of mice of different strains. Int J Cancer 22:487–494.

Potten CS. 1975. Epidermal cell production rates. J Invest Dermatol 65:488–500.

Raick AN. 1974. Cell proliferation and promoting action in skin carcinogenesis. Cancer Res 34:920–926.

Reiners JJ, Slaga TJ. 1983. Effects of tumor promoters on the rate and commitment to terminal differentiation of subpopulations of murine keratinocytes. Cell 32:247–255.

Reiners JJ, Nesnow S, Slaga TJ. 1984. Murine susceptibility to two-stage carcinogenesis is influenced by the agent used for promotion. Carcinogenesis 5:301–307.

Sisskin EE, Gray T, Barrett JC 1982. Correlation between sensitivity to tumor promotion and sustained hyperplasia of mice and rats treated with 12-0-tetradecanoylphorbol-13-acetate. Carcinogenesis 3:403–407.

Slaga TJ. 1983. Cellular and molecular mechanisms of tumour promotion. Cancer Surveys 2(4):595–612.

Slaga TJ, Fischer SM. 1983. Strain differences and solvent effects in mouse skin carcinogenesis experiments using carcinogens, tumor initiators and promoters. In Hamburger F, ed., Progress in Experimental Tumor Research, vol. 26. S. Karger, Basel, pp. 85–109.

Slaga TJ, Klein-Szanto AJP. 1983. Initiation-promotion versus complete skin carcinogenesis in mice: Importance of dark basal keratinocytes (stem cells). Cancer Invest 1:425–436.

Slaga TJ, Fischer SM, Weeks CE, Klein-Szanto AJP. 1981. Cellular and biochemical mechanisms of mouse skin tumor promoters. In Hodgson E, Bend J, Philpot RM, eds., Reviews in Biochemical Toxicology, vol 3. Elsevier North-Holland, Inc., New York, pp. 231–281.

Slaga TJ, Fischer SM, Weeks CE, Klein-Szanto AJP, Reiners J. 1982. Studies on the mechanisms involved in multistage carcinogenesis in mouse skin. J Cell Biochem 18:99–119.

Trosko JE, Yotti LP, Warren ST, Tsushimoto G, Chang CC. 1982. Inhibition of cell-cell communication by tumor promoters, In Hecker E, ed., Cocarcinogenesis and Biological Effects of Tumor Promoters. Raven Press, New York, pp. 565–585.

Van Duuren BL, Sivak A, Katz C, Seidman J, Melchionne S. 1975. The effect of aging and interval between primary and secondary treatment in two stage carcinogenesis on mouse skin. Cancer Res 35:502–505.

Varshavsky A. 1981. Phorbol ester dramatically increases incidence of methotrexate-resistant mouse cells: Possible mechanisms and relevance to tumor promotion. Cell 25:561–572.

Wilson VL, Jones PA. 1983. Inhibition of DNA methylation by chemical carcinogens in vitro. Cell 32:239.

Yuspa SH, Morgan DL. 1981. Mouse skin cells resistant to terminal differentiation associated with initiation of carcinogenesis. Nature 293:72–74.

Yuspa SH, Hennings H, Kulsease-Martin M, Lichti U. 1982. The study of tumor promotion in a cell culture model for mouse skin. In Hecker E, ed., Cocarcinogenesis and Biological Effects of Tumor Promoters. Raven Press, New York, pp. 217–230.

Symposium on Fundamental Cancer Research, Vol. 39.
© 1987 by The University of Texas System Cancer Center.

4. Role of Oncogenes and Tumor Suppressor Genes in a Multistep Model of Carcinogenesis

J. Carl Barrett, Mitsuo Oshimura, and Minoru Koi

Environmental Carcinogenesis Group, National Institute of Environmental Health Sciences, Research Triangle Park, North Carolina 27709

We demonstrated previously that carcinogen-induced neoplastic transformation of Syrian hamster embryo (SHE) cells requires multiple steps. Normal, diploid SHE cells and carcinogen-induced preneoplastic cells were transfected with different oncogenes. The normal, early-passage cells were not transformed by the v-Ha-*ras* or v-*myc* oncogenes alone, but the two oncogenes combined caused tumors in nude mice and syngeneic hamsters. Cytogenetic analysis of the *ras*-plus-*myc*-induced tumors showed a nonrandom chromosome loss (monosomy of chromosome 15) in the *ras/myc* tumor cells. Tumorigenicity of the *ras/myc* tumor cells was suppressed following hybridization with normal SHE cells; reexpression of tumorigenicity at later passages correlated with loss of chromosome 15. The hybrid cells in which tumorigenicity was suppressed still expressed the *ras* and *myc* oncogenes.

An early change in carcinogen-induced neoplastic progression of SHE cells is induction of immortality. At early passages, immortal cells retain the ability to suppress tumorigenicity in cell hybrids. This ability decreases with passaging of immortal cell lines. The susceptibility of immortal cell lines to neoplastic transformation by DNA transfection with the v-Ha-*ras* oncogene or tumor DNA inversely correlated with the tumor-suppressive ability of the cells in cell hybrids. These observations indicate that neoplastic transformation of SHE cells involves at least three steps: (1) induction of immortality, (2) activation of a transforming gene or oncogene, and (3) loss of or inactivation of a tumor-suppressor gene.

There is considerable research interest in positive, growth stimulatory factors in carcinogenesis because of our increasing understanding of oncogenes and autocrine growth factors (Sporn and Roberts 1985). Yet, evidence also exists for negative regulatory factors in carcinogenesis including (1) numerous examples of reversion of the malignant state to the nonmalignant state by altering the environment or treatment of tumor cells with certain chemicals or differentiation inducing substances, (2) suppression of tumorigenicity in cell hybrids, and (3) studies of genetic predisposition to cancer in humans and animals (Barrett 1987). With the increasing evidence that carcinogenesis is a multistep process (Farber et al. 1987), it may be possible to understand how an interaction between multiple positive and negative regulatory changes contribute to the carcinogenic process.

In this chapter, we will present recent findings on the genetic changes involved in the multistep process of neoplastic development of Syrian hamster embryo (SHE) cells in culture following either carcinogenic treatment or transfection with viral oncogenes. These studies suggest that activation of positive factors (oncogenes) and loss of negative growth regulatory functions (tumor-suppressor genes) are necessary and distinct changes in neoplastic progression.

MULTISTEP NEOPLASTIC PROGRESSION OF SYRIAN HAMSTER EMBRYO CELLS IN CULTURE

For a number of years, we have been studying the mechanisms of carcinogen-induced neoplastic progression of SHE cells in culture (Barrett and Ts'o 1978). This system has a number of advantages, including the use of cells with a stable, diploid karyotype, a low incidence of spontaneous transformation but a high sensitivity to carcinogen-induced transformation, and existence of quantitative markers for early carcinogen-induced changes (Barrett et al. 1984). One of the important features of this system is that the neoplastic conversion of these cells requires a number of different steps, and phenotype markers exist to identify cells at different stages of neoplastic progression (Fig. 4.1).

Our studies indicate that following carcinogen treatment, neoplastic progression of these cells requires *at least* two identifiable changes: induction of immortality

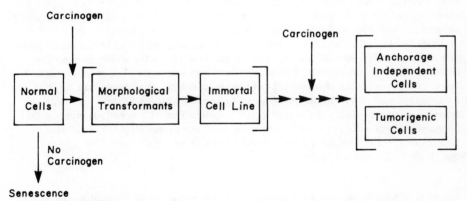

Figure 4.1 Neoplastic progression of Syrian hamster cells. Normal cells have a flat morphology and grow in an orderly array in parallel, swirling patterns. If subcultured for 10–20 passages (30–40 population doublings), the normal cells enlarge and cease proliferation (termed cellular senescence). If exposed to a chemical carcinogen, colonies of cells are observed with an altered morphology (criss-crossed growth with cells piling on top of each other, increased basophilic and increased nuclear-cytoplasmic ratio). When isolated some of these colonies escape cellular senescence and grow indefinitely (termed immortality). These cells are nontumorigenic at this time but, after further growth, give rise to new variant cells that grow in soft agar and produce tumors when injected into nude mice or syngeneic hamsters. The immortal cells have an increased propensity to develop into tumorigenic cells and hence the immortal cell population is termed intermediate or preneoplastic. The number of passages required to convert immortal cells to tumor cells is variable, and this process can sometimes be accelerated by secondary carcinogenic exposure.

and neoplastic conversion of immortal cells (Barrett and Fletcher 1987). This pattern of neoplastic transformation with chemical carcinogens is strikingly parallel to the findings that two cooperating oncogenes, *ras* plus *myc*, are required for neoplastic conversion of primary rat cells and with the hypothesis that these two oncogenes influence immortality and neoplastic conversion, respectively (Land et al. 1983, Ruley 1983). In fact, we have demonstrated that the v-Ha-*ras* plus v-*myc* oncogenes together, but not alone, neoplastically transform the SHE cells (Thomassen et al. 1985).

We have attempted to define the changes in the oncogenes involved in chemical carcinogen–induced immortality and subsequent neoplastic conversion of the immortal cells. Although we have not identified any specific oncogenes activated in the carcinogen-induced immortal cells, we have shown that a nonrandom chromosome change (trisomy of chromosome 11) occurs in some immortal cell lines (Oshimura et al. 1986). Morphological transformation and immortality are induced in these cells by chemicals which induce numerical changes in the absence of detectable gene mutations (Barrett et al. 1985), results that are consistent with an important role for aneuploidy in this step.

In contrast to the conclusions of others (Land et al. 1983, Ruley 1983), we do not have evidence that the v-*myc* oncogene directly induces immortality of the SHE cells. Cells transfected with v-*myc* plus v-Ha-*ras* oncogenes are neoplastically transformed (Thomassen et al, 1985). However, colonies of cells containing the v-Ha-*ras* and v-*myc* oncogenes are not initially immortal but rather undergo crisis and only a rare subpopulation escapes senescence to yield an immortal cell line (Annab L, Gilmer T, Barrett JC, unpublished data). The observed immortality of rat cells transfected with *myc* oncogenes may relate to the higher spontaneous rate of escape fron senescence observed with rat versus hamster cells (Barrett and Fletcher 1987). Neither have we observed induction of immortality or neoplastic conversion by transfection of the cells with an EJ-*ras* oncogene linked to two transcriptional enhancers in contrast to the reported findings of others (Spandidos and Wilkie 1984). Cotransfection of the SHE cells, however, with this *ras* gene modified with various enhancer elements plus v-*myc* results in tumors that grow more rapidly than tumors induced by v-Ha-*ras* plus v-*myc* oncogenes (Annab L, Barrett JC, unpublished data).

Analysis of carcinogen-induced tumorigenic cells for transforming genes in the NIH 3T3 transfection assay has yielded positive results in about 50% of the cell lines examined to date. Tumor cells derived from cultures treated with benzo(a)pyrene, asbestos, or diethylstilbestrol are positive in this assay, and preliminary characterization of the secondary foci indicates the presence of an activated *ras* oncogene with a mutation in the twelfth codon (Gilmer T, Annab L, Barrett JC, unpublished data). These activated *ras* genes are observed in the tumor cells but not the immortal, nontumorigenic cells, a finding consistent with *ras* activation's being a late, postimmortalization step.

Although the two steps of immortalization and neoplastic transformation are involved in carcinogen-induced neoplastic development, certain observations suggest that additional changes are also needed (Barrett et al. 1987). For example, not all immortal cell lines respond the same; some readily progress to the tumorigenic state either spontaneously or following treatment with carcinogens or viral oncogenes, whereas other cell lines are refractory to induction of neoplastic transformation by these treatments.

THE ROLE OF LOSS OF TUMOR SUPPRESSOR GENE IN NEOPLASTIC TRANSFORMATION OF SHE CELLS

Data from two lines of study in our laboratory have led us to the conclusion that the loss of a tumor suppressive function or gene is a key step in the progression of these cells. These data will be discussed in the next two sections.

Nonrandom Loss of Chromosome 15 in Syrian Hamster Tumors Induced by v-Ha-*ras* Plus v-*myc* Oncogenes

Neoplastic transformation of SHE cells by two cooperating oncogenes, v-Ha-*ras* plus v-*myc,* is consistent with a multistep model of carcinogenesis. However, the number of steps necessary to convert a normal cell into a malignant cell is unknown. If activation of two oncogenes is sufficient for tumorigenicity, tumors derived from diploid cells transformed by the transfected oncogenes may remain diploid or have only random chromosome alterations. Therefore, we examined the karotypes of tumors formed after transfection of SHE cells with v-Ha-*ras* plus v-*myc* oncogenes (Oshimura et al. 1985). We observed that tumors induced by v-Ha-*ras* plus v-*myc* were monoclonal and had a nonrandom chromosome change, monosomy of chromosome 15. This chromosome loss was found in six of six *ras/ myc* tumors examined but not in polyoma-induced tumors. Thus, an additional change, loss of chromosome 15, is advantageous or required for tumorigenicity induced by v-Ha-*ras* plus v-*myc* oncogenes.

In order to clarify the role of monosomy 15 in the expression of the tumorigenicity of the cells derived from the v-Ha-*ras* plus v-*myc*–induced tumors (*ras/myc*–T cells), we made hybrids between these tumor cells and normal SHE cells. The results of these studies are summarized in Figure 4.2 (Oshimura et al. 1987). One surprising finding was that over half of the cell hybrids that formed became senescent after isolation (<20 population doublings). This did not appear to be a consequence of toxicity from the fusion procedure, since the hybrid colonies grew vigorously at first. Rather, we interpret this finding to indicate that immortality is recessive in hamster × hamster hybrids as has been reported in human × human hybrids (Pereira-Smith and Smith 1983).

The SHE × *ras/myc*–T hybrids that became senescent could not be examined directly for tumorigenicity, but presumably these cells were nontumorigenic. Consistent with this suggestion is our observation that none of the hybrid cells that formed immediately after fusion had the ability to grow in soft agar. When we analyzed the hybrid cells that escaped cellular senescence, we found that the tumorigenicity and anchorage-independent growth ability of these cells were totally lost or greatly reduced when compared with the parental *ras/myc* tumor cells. Karotypic analysis of these hybrid cells showed that they contained three copies of chromo-

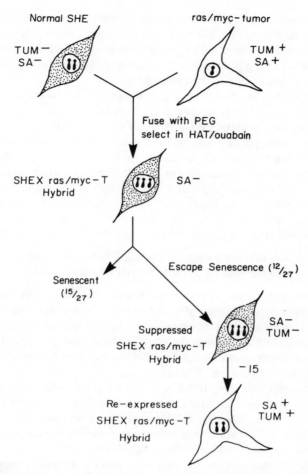

Figure 4.2. Suppression and reexpression of tumorigenicity and anchorage-independent growth in hybrids between normal Syrian hamster embryo (SHE) cells and *ras/myc*-tumor cells. A cell line derived from tumor induced by transfection of SHE cells with v-Ha-*ras* plus v-*myc* oncogenes was made resistant to 6-thioguanine and ouabain. These cells were fused with SHE cells by treatment with polyethylglycol (PEG), and the hybrids were selected in media containing HAT and ouabain (Koi and Barrett 1986). The resultant hybrid cells were unable to grow on soft agar but grew on plastic. When large colonies (>1000 cells) growing on plastic were isolated, >50% of the colonies became senescent. The colonies which escaped senescence were still non-tumorigenic (TUM⁻) and failed to grow on agar (SA⁻). These suppressed SHE × *ras/myc*-T hybrids contained three copies of chromosome 15 (two from the parental SHE cells and one from the parental *ras/myc*-T cells, which are monosomic for this chromosome). After further growth in culture, rare variants arose in the culture that were tumorigenic (TUM⁺) and grew in agar (SA⁺). Isolation and karyotypic analysis of these variants revealed that they had lost a single copy of chromosome 15, but no other nonrandom chromosome changes were observed.

some 15, as would be expected for a hybrid between a normal diploid cell and a tumor cell with monosomy 15. The nontumorigenic SHE × *ras/myc*–T hybrids still expressed RNA which hybridized to the viral *ras* and *myc* genes and high levels of the mutated form of the p21^{ras} protein. Thus, suppression of tumorigenicity was not due to the lack of expression of the oncogenes.

When the hybrid cells were passaged, anchorage-independent and tumorigenic variant cells arose at a low frequency in the population. These cells were cloned, and comparisons were made of the karotypes of the parental cells, hybrids that were suppressed for tumorigenicity and anchorage independence, and hybrids that re-expressed these phenotypes. These studies revealed that the suppressed hybrids contained the chromosome complement of both parental cells as anticipated. The hybrids that reexpressed tumorigenicity had lost only a few chromosomes; a non-random loss of chromosome 15, but no other nonrandom chromosome loss, was observed. These results suggest that the loss of chromosome 15 results in the loss of a cellular gene that effects a phenotype necessary for neoplastic transformation.

Loss of Tumor Suppressor Function during Chemically Induced Neoplastic Progression of Syrian Hamster Embryo Cells

The cell hybrid experiments described above were performed with tumor cells induced by oncogene transfection. We also have examined the suppression of tumorigenicity of chemically transformed cells in cell hybrids with normal early passage SHE cells and determined the stage in the multistep neoplastic process at which this tumor suppression function is lost (Koi and Barrett 1986).

Cell hybrids between normal, SHE cells, and a highly tumorigenic, chemically transformed hamster cell line, BP6T-M3, were formed, selected, and analyzed. Like the SHE × *ras/myc*–T hybrids, approximately 50% of the BP6T × SHE hybrids became senescent. When the hybrids that did not become senescent were analyzed, tumorigenicity and anchorage-independent growth were suppressed. These two phenotypes segregated coordinately in these cells.

To determine at what stage in the neoplastic process the tumor suppression that was observed in the normal SHE cells was lost, two chemically induced immortal cell lines (DES-4 and 10W) at different passages were fused to BP6T cells. When DES-4 × BP6T hybrids were assayed for growth in agar, a significant suppression (500- to 5,000-fold) of anchorage-independent growth was observed. Likewise, the tumorigenicity or tumor latency of the hybrids was suppressed. However, a different pattern was observed in 10W × BP6T hybrids compared to DES-4 × 10W hybrids. All of the 10W × BP6T hybrids grew in agar with a frequency from >1% to 46% (only a 2- to 50-fold reduction). These hybrids were also much more tumorigenic; the tumor latency period was, in some cases, equal to BP6T parental cells and was increased to 13 days, at most.

To confirm the differences between 10W cells and DES-4 cells in terms of their abilities to suppress anchorage-independent growth of BP6T cells in hybrids, a direct assay of anchorage-independent growth of hybrids was performed (Table 4.1). In this assay the cells of interest were fused and after a 24-hour recovery period, the

Table 4.1 *Suppression/Expression of Anchorage-Independent Phenotype in Hybrids of BP6T-M3 Cells and Various Other Cells*

Cell Line Fused to BP6T-M3 Cells	Hybrid Frequency[a] ($\times 10^{-4}$)	ag$^+$ Hybrid Frequency[b] ($\times 10^{-4}$)	Ratio of ag$^+$ Frequency to Total Hybrid Frequency
BP6T	35.2	37.9	1.076
SHE (p5)	7.9	0.007	0.0009
10W (p5)	17.6	0.005	0.0003
10W (p15)	9.9	7.08	0.715
DES-4 (p35)	25.6	0.054	0.0021
DES-4 (p58)	22.4	1.39	0.062

Data from Koi and Barrett 1986.
[a] Hybrid frequency was determined from the number of colonies growing on plastic dishes in HAT/ouabain medium two weeks after selection.
[b] Ag$^+$ hybrid frequency was determined from the number of colonies growing in agar containing selective (HAT/ouabain) medium at three weeks after selection.

hybrids were isolated in selective medium either on plastic or directly in agar with selective medium. The ratio of hybrids growing in agar (ag$^+$) to total hybrids is therefore a measure of the cells' ability to suppress anchorage-independent growth. Control experiments with BP6T $\times$ BP6T-m3 hybrids resulted in the same number of hybrids in agar and on plastic (ratio = 1.076) (Table 4.1), while the ratio was reduced to 0.0009 for SHE $\times$ BP6T hybrids. 10W cells at passage 15 reduced the ratio of ag$^+$ hybrids to total hybrids to only 0.711. However, at an earlier passage (p5) the 10W cells were still effective in suppressing anchorage-independent growth (ratio = 0.0003). Hybrids of 10W (p5) $\times$ BP6T cells growing on plastic were isolated and analyzed for anchorage-independent growth; all were suppressed for this phenotype.

When DES-4 cells at passage 35 and passage 58 were fused with BP6T cells, the ratio of ag$^+$ hybrids to total hybrids was 0.0021 and 0.062, respectively. Therefore, at the later passage, the ability of the cells to suppress anchorage independence decreased but not to the degree observed with 10W cells. Subclones of 10W cells (p15) and DES-4 cells (p58) were randomly isolated and tested for the ability to suppress anchorage-independent growth of BP6T cells. These subclones were heterogeneous in their ability to suppress tumorigenicity in cell hybrids; some clones retained the tumor suppression ability but others had lost this function (Koi and Barrett, 1986).

In order to determine if the cells with differing abilities to suppress anchorage-independent growth differed in their susceptibility to transformation by DNA transfection, the cells were treated with BP6T genomic DNA or v-Ha-*ras* plasmid DNA by the calcium phosphate–transfection method, and after five days they were assayed for anchorage-independent growth and tumorigenicity. When the cells were transfected with v-Ha-*ras* DNA, 10W cells, which are not effective in suppressing tumorigenicity and anchorage-independent growth (sup$^-$), grew in soft agar with 1000-fold higher frequency than DES-4 (sup$^+$) cells (Table 4.2). This difference was

Table 4.2. *Susceptibility of Immortal Cells to Transfection by Different DNAs*

Recipient Cells[a]	Phenotypes[b]	G418^r Colonies[c] with pSV2neo	Agar Colonies[d] with v-Ha-*ras*	Agar Colonies[d] with BP6T DNA
DES-4	tum$^-$, ag$^-$, sup$^+$	3×10^{-3}	2.5×10^{-6}	$< 1 \times 10^{-6}$
10W	tum$^-$, ag$^-$, sup$^-$	9×10^{-4}	3.8×10^{-3}	54×10^{-6}

[a] DES-4 p55; 10W p15.
[b] Cells failed to form tumors in nude mice (tum$^-$) or grow in agar (ag$^-$) when 10^6 cells were assayed. Cells either suppress (sup$^+$) or fail to suppress (sup$^-$) tumorigenicity and anchorage-independent growth of BP6T cells hybridization.
[c] Cells transfected with pSV2neo as described (Thomassen et al. 1984). Data expressed in colonies per microgram of DNA transfected.
[d] Cells were transfected with v-Ha-*ras* (Thomassen et al. 1984) or BP6T DNA (Koi and Barrett 1986) selected 3–5 days later for growth in agar.

unrelated to the efficiency of uptake and expression of DNA, since the frequency of G418^r colonies following transfection with pSV2-neo was slightly greater for DES-4 cells (Table 4.2).

SIGNIFICANCE OF TUMOR SUPPRESSOR GENES IN A MULTISTEP MODEL OF CARCINOGENESIS

Based upon our results, we propose the hypothesis that chemically induced neoplastic progression of SHE cells involves at least three steps (Table 4.3). The lines of evidence supporting this model are summarized in Table 4.4. The possibility exists that the induction of immortality involves two steps, activation of a proto-oncogene and loss of a senescence function or gene. In the absence of mapping this function to a specific chromosome, the existence of a senescence gene remains speculative.

The finding of the tumor-suppressive function associated with the loss of a specific chromosome in the *ras/myc* tumor cells strongly supports the existence of a specific tumor suppressor gene on this chromosome. As summarized in Table 4.5, other cell hybrid studies have shown an association with the loss of a specific chromosome and re-expression of tumorigenicity in suppressed hybrids. Recently, Saxon and coworkers (1986) have shown in very elegant and convincing experiments that human chromosome 11 can suppress tumorigenicity in hybrids of normal human fibroblasts and HeLa cells.

The number of tumor suppressor genes in a cell is unknown, but it is reasonable to assume, on the basis of available data, that a family of these genes exists. At least 50 dominantly inherited cancer susceptibilities have been identified in humans (Mulvihill 1971). In none of these human cancer susceptibilities has a mutation of a proto-oncogene been implicated; rather, mutations in a different class of genes, tumor suppression genes, appear to be inherited in these individuals (Knudson 1985). Individuals who inherit a heterozygous, germ-line mutation in one of these genes are predisposed to develop specific cancers (e.g., Wilms' tumor and retinoblas-

Table 4.3. *Genetic Events in Multistep Carcinogenesis of Syrian Hamster Embryo Cells*

1. Acquisition of immortality
   a. activation of proto-oncogene ("immortalization oncogene")
   b. loss of senescence function or gene
2. Activation of a second proto-oncogene ("transforming oncogene")
3. Loss or inactivation of tumor suppressor gene

Note: These genetic events may arise in any sequence.

Table 4.4. *Evidence for a Role of Tumor-Suppressor Genes in Neoplastic Transformation of Syrian Hamster Embryo Cells*

1. Tumorigenicity and anchorage-independent growth are recessive traits in hybrids between tumorigenic cells and normal Syrian hamster embryo cells.
2. Cells neoplastically transformed by transfection with v-Ha-*ras* plus v-*myc* oncogenes have a nonrandom loss of chromosome 15.
3. Hybrids between *ras/myc* tumor cells and normal Syrian hamster embryo cells are suppressed for tumorigenicity even though they express the activated oncogenes.
4. Carcinogen-induced immortal cell lines at early passages retain the ability to suppress tumorigenicity in cell hybrids, and this ability is lost as the cells are passaged.
5. Subclones of immortal cells are heterogeneous for the ability to suppress tumorigenicity in cell hybrids; some retain this ability (sup+) while others have lost it (sup−).
6. sup+ cells are refractory or less sensitive than sup− cells to neoplastic conversion by v-Ha-*ras* oncogene, BP6T tumor DNA, and mutagens.
7. The majority of hybrids between immortal and normal Syrian hamster embryo cells became senescent indicating that senescence is dominant over immortality (senescence gene?).

Table 4.5. *Chromosomes That Have Been Proposed to Carry Suppressor Genes for Tumorigenicity, Anchorage-Independent Growth, or Both Based on Cell Hybrid Studies*

Tumorigenic Parental Cell	Nontumorigenic Parental Cell	Chromosome(s) with Possible Suppressor Gene	Reference
Mouse melanoma, carcinoma, lymphoma, or sarcoma	Normal mouse fibroblasts	Mouse #4	Evans et al. (1982) Cowell & Franks (1984)
Chinese hamster fibrosarcoma	Normal human fibroblasts	Human #2,9,10,1,17	Klinger & Shows (1983)
Human carcinoma (HeLa)	Normal human fibroblasts	Human #11,14	Stanbridge et al. (1981)
Human HT1080 fibrosarcoma	Normal human fibroblasts	Human #1,4	Benedict et al. (1984)
Syrian hamster BHK sarcoma	Normal human fibroblasts	Human #1	Stoler & Bouck (1985)
Syrian hamster *ras/myc* fibrosarcoma	Syrian hamster embryo cells	Syrian hamster #15	Oshimura et al. (1985)

toma). In these cancers, the locus of the inherited mutation frequently becomes homozygous or hemizygous by a variety of secondary chromosomal mutations (Cavenee et al. 1983). The implication of these findings is that these genes suppress the expression of the cancer unless a mutation or a deletion of both alleles of the gene arises. Different tumor suppressor genes are apparently involved in different tumors since genetic predispositions are mapped to different chromosomal localizations (e.g., chromosome 1 in neuroblastoma, chromosome 11 in Wilms' tumor, and chromosome 13 in retinoblastoma). However, the same tumor suppressor gene may be involved in histologically different tumors. Involvement of chromosome 11 is observed in Wilms' tumor and bladder carcinomas (Koufos et al. 1984, Fearon et al. 1985), and the hereditary predisposition to one type of tumor is shared with other specific tumor types. For example, retinoblastoma and osteosarcoma incidences are both increased in affected individuals (Murphree and Benedict 1984).

In *Drosophila melanogaster,* at least 24 recessive genes that are associated with tissue-specific tumors when mutated have been identified (Gateff 1978). One of these genes (lethal (2) giant larvae) recently has been cloned (Mechler et al. 1985). When the normal allele of this gene is transposed into *D. melanogaster* with a mutant allele of this gene, the development of tumors in these flies is suppressed (Mechler BM, personal communication, 1986). Further studies of these *D. melanogaster* genes should help elucidate the nature of the homologous mammalian genes and facilitate their cloning.

Our data show that both the inactivation of tumor suppressor genes and the activation of proto-oncogenes are important steps in neoplastic development of SHE cells. Cells that retain the tumor-suppressive function are not tumorigenic, even when expressing activated oncogenes; conversely, cells that have lost this tumor-suppressive function but do not have an activated oncogene are nontumorigenic. Hence, loss of the suppressor gene function alone is insufficient for tumor growth. In addition to the tumor suppressor gene that is still active in some immortal cell lines, a cellular senescence gene may also have to be lost for neoplastic development. This may represent another type of tumor suppressor gene. Thus, the multistep nature of carcinogenesis is possibly attributable to the need to affect both classes of genes (oncogenes and tumor-suppressor genes) involved in tumor development.

Many areas of future research in tumor suppressor genes are evident. The cloning of these genes and elucidation of their normal functions will undoubtedly reveal unexpected findings. It will be important to identify the number and functions of these genes. In addition, it will be interesting to determine whether the inactivation of specific tumor suppressor genes correlates with the activation of specific proto-oncogenes in different tumor types. The stages of in vivo neoplastic development at which these genes are lost or inactivated and the mechanisms by which chemical carcinogens, tumor promoters, or both affect the function of these genes are also key areas of study in chemical carcinogenesis.

REFERENCES

Barrett JC. 1987. Genetic and epigenetic mechanisms in carcinogenesis. *In* Barrett JC, ed., Mechanisms of Environmental Carcinogenesis: Role of Genetic and Epigenetic Changes, vol. I. CRC Press, Boca Raton (in press).

Barrett JC, Fletcher WF. 1987. Cellular and molecular mechanisms of multistep carcinogenesis in cell culture models. *In* Barrett JC, ed., Mechanisms of Environmental Carcinogenesis: Multistep Models of Carcinogenesis, vol. II, CRC Press, Boca Raton (in press).

Barrett JC, Hesterberg TW, Thomassen DG. 1984. Use of cell transformation systems for carcinogenicity testing and mechanistic studies of carcinogenesis. Pharmacol Rev 36: 53S–70S.

Barrett JC, Hesterberg TW, Oshimura M, Tsutsui T. 1985. Role of chemically induced mutagenic events in neoplastic transformation of Syrian hamster embryo cells. *In* Barrett JC, Tennant RW, eds., Mammalian Cell Transformation: Mechanisms of Carcinogenesis and Assays for Carcinogenes, vol. 9. Raven Press, New York, pp. 123–138.

Barrett JC, Koi M, Gilmer TM, Oshimura M. 1987. Oncogene and chemical-induced neoplastic progression: Role of tumor suppression. J Cell Biochem (in press).

Barrett JC, Ts'o POP. 1978. Evidence for the progressive nature of neoplastic transformation in vitro. Proc Natl Acad Sci USA 75:3761–3765.

Benedict WF, Weissman BE, Mark C, Stanbridge EJ. 1984. Tumorigenicity in nude mice of hybrids between the human fibrosarcoma cell line HT-1080 and normal human fibroblasts is gene dose dependent. Cancer Res 44:3471–3478.

Cavenee WK, Dryja TP, Phillips RA, et al. 1983. Expression of recessive alleles by chromosomal mechanisms in retinoblastoma. Nature 305:779–784.

Cowell JK, Franks LM. 1984. The ability of normal mouse cells to reduce the malignant potential of transformed mouse bladder epithelial cells depend on their somatic origin. Int J Cancer 33:657–667.

Evans EP, Burtenshaw MD, Brown BB, Hennion R, Harris H. 1982. The analysis of malignancy by cell fusion. IX. Re-examination and clarification of the cytogenetic problem. J Cell Sci 56:113–130.

Farber E, Rotstein JB, Eriksson LC. 1987. Cancer development as a multistep process: Experimental studies in animals. *In* Barrett JC, ed., Mechanisms of Environmental Carcinogenesis: Multistep Models of Carcinogenesis, vol. II. CRC Press, Boca Raton (in press).

Fearon ER, Feinberg AP, Hamilton SH, Vogelstein B. 1985. Loss of genes on the short arm of chromosome 11 in bladder cancer. Nature 318:377–380.

Gateff E. 1978. Malignant neoplasms of genetic origin in *Drosophilia melanogaster.* Science 200:1448–1459.

Klinger HP, Shows TB. 1983. Suppression of tumorigenicity in somatic cell hybrids. II. Human chromosomes implicated as suppressors of tumorigenicity in hybrids with Chinese hamster ovary cells. JNCI 71:559–569.

Koufos A, Hansen MF, Lampkin DB, et al. 1984. Loss of alleles at loci on human chromosome 11 during genesis of Wilms' tumour. Nature 309:170–172.

Knudson AG Jr. 1985. Hereditary cancer, oncogenes, and antioncogenes. Cancer Res 45: 1437–1443.

Koi M, Barrett JC. 1986. Loss of tumor suppression function during chemically induced neoplastic progression of Syrian hamster embryo cells. Proc Natl Acad Sci USA 83: 5992–5996.

Land H, Parada LF, Weinberg RA. 1983. Tumorigenic conversion of primary embryo fibroblasts requires at least two cooperating oncogenes. Nature 304:596–602.

Mechler BM, McGinnis W, Gehring WJ. 1985. Molecular cloning of lethal(2)giant larvae, a recessive oncogene of Drosophilia melanogaster. EMBO J 4:1551–1557.

Murphree AL, Benedict WF. 1984. Retinoblastoma: Clues to human oncogenesis. Science 223:1028–1033.

Mulvihill JJ. 1971. Genetic repertory of human neoplasia. *In* Mulvihill JJ, Miller RW, Fraumeni JF, eds., Genetics of Human Cancer. Raven Press, New York, pp. 137–143.

Oshimura M, Gilmer TM, Barrett JC. 1985. Nonrandom loss of chromosome 15 in Syrian hamster tumors induced by v-Ha-*ras* plus v-*myc* oncogenes. Nature 316:636–639.

Oshimura M, Hesterberg TW, Barrett JC. 1986. An early, non-random karyotypic change in immortal Syrian hamster cell lines transformed by asbestos: trisomy of chromosome 11. Cancer Genet Cytogenet 22:225–237.

Pereira-Smith OM, Smith JR. 1983. Evidence for the recessive nature of cellular immortality. Science 221:963–966.

Ruley HE. 1983. Adenovirus early region 1A enables viral and cellular transforming genes to transform primary cells in culture. Nature 304:602–609.

Saxon PJ, Srivatsan ES, Stanbridge EJ. 1986. Introduction of human chromosome 11 via microcell transfer controls tumorigenic expression of HeLa cells. EMBO J (in press).

Spandidos DA, Wilkie NM. 1984. Malignant transformation of early passage rodent cells by a single mutated human oncogene. Nature 310:469–475.

Sporn MB, Roberts AB. 1985. Autocrine growth factors and cancer. Nature 213:745–750.

Stanbridge EJ, Flandemeyer RR, Daniels FW, Nelson-Rees WA. 1981. Specific chromosome loss associated with the expression of tumorigenicity in human cell hybrids. Somatic Cell Mol Genet 7:699–712.

Stoler A, Bouck N. 1985. Identification of a single chromosome in the normal human genome essential for suppression of hamster cell transformation. Proc Natl Acad Sci USA 82:570–574.

Thomassen DG, Gilmer TM, Annab LA, Barrett JC. 1985. Evidence for multiple steps in neoplastic transformation of normal and preneoplastic Syrian hamster embryo cells following transfection with Harvey murine sarcoma virus oncogene (v-Ha-*ras*). Cancer Res 45:726–732.

TRANSGENIC EXPRESSION

Symposium on Fundamental Cancer Research, Vol. 39.
© 1987 by The University of Texas System Cancer Center.

5. Retroviruses as Tools for Mammalian Development

Rudolf Jaenisch and Philippe Soriano

*Whitehead Institute for Biomedical Research and Department of Biology,
Massachusetts Institute of Technology, Cambridge, Massachusetts 02142*

Retroviruses have been used as probes for the study of mammalian development. Successful applications of this tool include (1) genetic labeling of cells for lineage studies in preimplantation and postimplantation development, (2) tagging important chromosomal regions of the mouse genome, (3) identifying genes that are expressed during early development, and (4) generating mutant mouse strains by insertional mutations that allow for molecular and functional analyses of developmental genes.

The introduction of foreign DNA sequences into mouse embryos and the generation of transgenic mice represents a powerful tool with which to probe into mammalian development because it combines a genetic and a molecular approach. In this approach, either mouse zygotes are microinjected with recombinant DNA (reviewed in Palmiter and Brinster 1985) or mouse embryos are exposed to retroviruses at different stages of development (Jaenisch et al. 1975, 1981, 1983, Jaenisch 1976, 1980). Retroviruses have been used as a tool for approaching a number of problems that are relevant to mammalian development and that, so far, have not been amenable to experimental analysis. They include the generation of developmental mutations by insertional mutagenesis, the analysis of lineage relationships in early mouse development, and the discovery of a high rate of unequal crossing-over events in meiosis. In this chapter, we will summarize briefly the interactions of retroviruses with the developing mouse embryo and the generation of some 50 transgenic mouse strains carrying a single provirus in the germ line at distinct chromosomal loci. We then will briefly summarize what is known about activation and chromosomal localization of the provirus and virus-induced insertional mutations in particular strains.

INSERTION OF MOLONEY LEUKEMIA VIRUSES INTO THE GERM LINE OF MICE

Mouse strains, termed Mov substrains, carrying a single Moloney leukemia proviral copy (Mo-MuLV) as a Mendelian determinant, were derived by exposing mouse embryos to infectious virus at different developmental stages.

Approximately 45 transgenic mouse strains carrying either the wild-type Mo-

Table 5.1. *Transgenic Mouse Strains Carrying a Moloney Leukemia Provirus in the Germ Line*

Mov Locus	Development of Viremia	Chromosomal Location	Phenotype	Reference
Mov-2,-4,-5,-6,-8, -11,-12,-23,-29,-30, -34,-35,-36	−	?	None	1,2
Mov-3,-16,-17,-18, -19,-20,-21,-22,-25, -27,-28,-37,-38,-39, -40,-41,-42,-43[a], -44[a],-45[a]	+	?	None	1,2
Mov-1	+	6	None	3,4
Mov-7	−	1	None	
Mov-9	+	11	None	
Mov-10	−	3	None	
Mov-14[b]	+	X	None	5
Mov-15	+	X/Y pairing reg.	None	6
Mov-24	+	Y	None	9
Mov-13[a]	+	11	Recessive lethal, α_1(I) collagen gene	4,7,8
Mov-34	−	?	Recessive lethal	9

References: 1. Jaenisch et al. 1981; 2. Soriano and Jaenisch 1986; 3. Breindl et al. 1979; 4. Müncke et al. 1986; 5. Stewart et al. 1983; 6. Harbers et al. 1986; 7. Jaenisch et al. 1983; 8. Schnieke et al. 1983; 9. Soriano et al. 1987.
[a] Embryos injected at the postimplantation stage.
[b] DNA microinjected into zygote pronucleus.

Table 5.2. *Transgenic Mouse Strains Carrying Recombinant Vectors in the Germ Line*

Mouse Strain	Transduced Gene	Expression
Gpt-1[a]	*E. coli gpt* gene	None
Glob-1[b]	Human β-globin gene	Hemopoietic tissues and muscle
	Bacterial *neo* gene	Muscle
Glob-2[b]	Human β-globin gene	Hemopoietic tissues
	Bacterial *neo* gene	None
Glob-3[b]	Human β-globin gene	Hemopoietic tissues
	Bacterial *neo* gene	None

[a] Jähner et al. 1985.
[b] Soriano et al. 1986.

MuLV or a modified provirus (Mo-MuLV[sup]) (Reik et al. 1985) have been derived from virus-infected preimplantation embryos (Jaenisch et al. 1981, Soriano and Jaenisch 1986), whereas four strains were derived from embryos microinjected with infectious virus at midgestation (Jaenisch 1980, Jaenisch et al. 1981, Soriano et al. 1987). Some known characteristics of these strains, including virus activation, chromosomal location, and mutant phenotype, are summarized in Table 5.1. Four strains have been derived by infection of embryos with recombinant retroviral vectors that transduced the bacterial *gpt* gene or the *neo* gene and the human β-globin gene into the germ line. The pattern of expression of the virus-transduced genes in these strains is summarized in Table 5.2.

EXPRESSION OF THE PROVIRAL GENOME IN MOV SUBSTRAINS OF MICE

Our initial efforts were aimed at analyzing retrovirus–host genome interactions during the course of mammalian development (reviewed in Jaenisch and Jähner 1984). Our findings can be summarized as follows: (1) A proviral genome inserted into the genome of the preimplantation embryo or into embryonal carcinoma cells will not be expressed. In contrast, virus microinjected into the embryo after implantation will replicate in cells of all tissues and will efficiently spread throughout the embryo (Jaenisch 1980, Jähner et al. 1982). (2) The block to virus expression, once established at the preimplantation stage, is maintained throughout later stages of development even at stages when the somatic cells have become competent to support viral replication. This suggested that transcriptional inactivity, once established at an early developmental stage, is maintained by a *cis*-acting mechanism. The development of viremia, which is seen in a number of strains (Jaenisch et al. 1981), is due to a rare event of virus activation in a small, unidentified population of cells. (3) Further work implicated DNA methylation in the maintenance, if not in the establishment, of gene inactivity (Stuhlmann et al. 1981, Harbers et al. 1981, Jähner and Jaenisch 1985a). Retroviruses become de novo methylated when introduced into preimplantation mouse embryos but not when introduced into postimplantation mouse embryos (Jähner et al. 1982). De novo methylase activity, as defined by these experiments, is characteristic of early embryonic cells and is not detected in cells of later developmental stages (Stewart et al. 1982, Gautsch and Wilson 1983). The activation of silent retroviral genomes by injection of 5-azacytidine into postnatal animals is consistent with the idea that DNA methylation has an important role in the maintenance of the transcriptional block (Jaenisch et al. 1985b). De novo methylation may not only be involved in activation of virus expression but may also be important for virus-induced repression of adjacent host genes.

TISSUE-SPECIFIC EXPRESSION OF GENES INTRODUCED INTO THE GERM LINE BY RETROVIRAL VECTORS

The evidence summarized above indicates that genes under the transcriptional control of the retroviral long terminal repeats are inactive when introduced into transgenic animals. However, when recombinant retroviral vectors carrying a complete genomic human β-globin gene, under the control of its own promoter, were introduced into the germ line, expression of the transduced gene in hematopoietic tissues was observed independently of the site of integration in the three transgenic mouse strains analyzed so far (Table 5.2) (Soriano et al. 1986). These observations indicate that transgenic animals that express the foreign gene in a tissue-specific manner can be generated by infection of mouse embryos with retroviral vectors.

PROVIRUS INSERTION INTO THE SEX CHROMOSOMES

In three mouse strains (Mov-14, -15, and -24), the provirus is transmitted in a sex chromosome–linked fashion. The most interesting results emerged from the genetic and molecular analyses of the Mov-15 strain (Harbers et al. 1986), which indicated that the provirus had integrated into the proximal part of the X/Y chromosome pseudoautosomal region. Proviral copies are lost or gained in 7% of all meioses in Mov-15 males, suggesting that unequal recombination events occur with high frequency in the pairing region. Mouse sequences flanking the proviruses were cloned and were shown to be tandemly repeated and highly polymorphic. These results demonstrate a useful application of genetically labeling a chromosomal region with a provirus. Only the presence of the unique proviral marker enabled us to measure the frequency of unequal crossing-over in a DNA region composed of repetitive sequences.

INDUCTION OF TWO INSERTIONAL MUTATIONS

To screen for recessive mutations induced by virus insertion, we have intercrossed mice heterozygous for approximately 50 different Mo-MuLV proviruses and identified homozygous offspring by Southern DNA analysis. For two integrations, designated as Mov-13 and Mov-34, we failed to obtain homozygous animals (see Table 5.1).

Our first mutant mouse strain, designated Mov-13, was obtained by microinjection of Moloney leukemia virus into postimplantation mouse embryos (Jaenisch et al. 1983). The virus insertion in this strain caused an embryonic recessive lethal mutation, with homozygous embryos dying at day 13 of gestation. The mutated gene was cloned and identified as coding for the αl chain of collagen I (Schnieke et al. 1983). This mouse strain was used to analyze the role of collagen in embryonic development (Löhler et al. 1984) and the molecular mechanisms involved in retrovirus-induced insertional mutagenesis. These experiments have been reviewed recently (Jaenisch et al. 1985a) and can be summarized as follows: the virus in the Mov-13 mouse strain has integrated into the first intron of the collagen gene (Harbers et al. 1984), resulting in a complete block of the developmentally regulated activation of collagen transcription. In vitro "run-off" transcription studies with isolated nuclei have shown that initiation of transcription is inhibited by the insertion (Hartung et al. 1986). Further molecular analyses demonstrated two virus-induced alterations of the mutated gene: first, the prevention of the appearance of a DNase I hypersensitive and transcription-associated site during development (Breindl et al. 1984) and second, de novo methylation of collagen sequences flanking the proviral insertion (Jähner and Jaenisch 1985b). Both compact chromatin conformation and methylation are associated with gene inactivity in many systems. De novo methylation of flanking mouse sequences has been induced not only by the

Mov-13 provirus but also by proviruses carried in other Mov strains. It is possible, therefore, that alterations in chromatin configuration and DNA methylation patterns are a common consequence of provirus insertion into the genome of embryonic cells and that these alterations are causally related to retrovirus-induced mutations.

Recently, we have identified a second virus-induced recessive lethal mutation. In contrast to Mov-13, the Mov-34 strain was derived from an embryo exposed to virus at the preimplantation stage (Table 5.1). Embryos homozygous for the proviral insertion at this locus die early after implantation. The cellular sequences flanking the provirus have been cloned with the help of the bacterial *sup* F gene, which is transduced by the virus (Reik et al. 1985). Our first analyses of the mutant locus indicate that no rearrangements of host sequences flanking the provirus have occurred, findings similar to ours with the Mov-13 mutant. Further experiments indicate that the virus has integrated close to a gene that is highly expressed in many cell types, including embryonal carcinoma cells. The available evidence indicates that the virus insertion blocks expression of this gene (Soriano et al. 1987).

CONCLUSIONS

Retroviruses have become an increasingly useful tool with which to probe molecular mechanisms of mammalian development. Successful applications of this tool include (1) genetic labeling of cells in the preimplantation (Soriano and Jaenisch 1986) and the postimplantation mouse embryo (Stuhlmann et al. 1984), allowing cell lineage studies, (2) the tagging of important chromosomal regions, which allows for genetic and molecular analyses (Harbers et al. 1986), (3) the identification of genes that are expressed in early embryonic cells (Barklis et al. 1986), and (4) the generation of insertional mutations that allows for molecular and functional analyses of genes important for embryonic development (Jaenisch et al. 1985a, Soriano et al. 1987). So far, the microinjection of DNA into the pronucleus has been the method of choice to achieve tissue-specific expression of genes in transgenic mice (Palmiter and Brinster 1985), while retrovirus-transduced genes under transcriptional control of the viral LTR are rarely or not at all expressed in the transgenic animal. To achieve tissue-specific expression, the retroviral vector–transduced genes may have to be placed under the control of internal promoters as demonstrated for the human β-globin gene (Soriano et al. 1986) (Table 5.2). Infection of embryos with retroviral vectors carrying genes under the control of internal promoters may, therefore, represent an alternative to the method of pronuclear DNA injection for deriving transgenic mice that express the foreign gene in a tissue-specific manner. Because retroviruses can be introduced efficiently into embryos at different stages, they permit manipulation of the embryo throughout development and thus are likely to become an increasingly important tool in experimental embryology.

ACKNOWLEDGMENT

This work was supported by grants HD-19105 from the National Institute of Health and PO1-CA 38497 from the National Cancer Institute.

REFERENCES

Barklis E, Mulligan R, Jaenisch R. 1986. Chromosomal position or virus mutation permits retrovirus expression in embryonal carcinoma cells. Cell 47:391–399.

Breindl M, Doehmer J, Willecke K, Dausman J, Jaenisch R. 1979. Germ line integration of Moloney leukemia virus: Identification of the chromosomal integration site. Proc Natl Acad Sci USA 76:1938–1942.

Breindl M, Harbers K, Jaenisch R. 1984. Retrovirus-induced lethal mutation in collagen I gene of mice is associated with altered chromatin structure. Cell 38:9–16.

Gautsch JW, Wilson MC. 1983. Delayed *de novo* methylation in teratocarcinoma suggests additional tissue-specific mechanisms for controlling gene expression. Nature 301:32–34.

Harbers K, Schnieke H, Stuhlmann D, Jähner D, Jaenisch R. 1981. DNA methylation and gene expression: Endogenous retroviral genome becomes infectious after molecular cloning. Proc Natl Acad Sci USA 78:7609–7613.

Harbers K, Kuehn M, Delius H, Jaenisch R. 1984. Insertion of retrovirus into the first intron of alpha 1(I) collagen gene leads to embryonic lethal mutation in mice. Proc Natl Acad Sci USA 81:1504–1508.

Harbers K, Soriano P, Muller U, Jaenisch J. 1986. High frequency of unequal recombination in the pseudoautosomal region revealed by proviral insertion in transgenic mouse strain. Nature 324:682–685.

Hartung S, Jaenisch R, Breindl M. 1986. Retrovirus insertion inactivates mouse αl(I) collagen by blocking initiation of transcription. Nature 320:365–367.

Jaenisch R. 1976. Germ line integration and Mendelian transmission of the exogenous Moloney leukemia virus. Proc Natl Acad Sci USA 73:1260–1264.

Jaenisch R. 1980. Retroviruses and embryogenesis: Microinjection of Moloney leukemia virus into midgestation mouse embryos. Cell 19:181–188.

Jaenisch R, Jähner D. 1984. Methylation, expression and chromosomal position of genes in mammals. Biochim Biophys Acta 782:1–9.

Jaenisch R, Fan H, Croker B. 1975. Infection of preimplantation mouse embryos and of newborn mice with leukemia virus: Tissue distribution of viral DNA and RNA and leukemogenesis in the adult animal. Proc Natl Acad Sci USA 72:4008–4012.

Jaenisch R, Jähner D, Nobis P, et al. 1981. Chromosomal position and activation of retroviral genomes inserted into the germ line of mice. Cell 24:515–529.

Jaenisch R, Harbers K. Schnieke A, et al. 1983. Germline integration of Moloney murine leukemia virus at the Mov13 locus leads to recessive lethal mutation and early embryonic death. Cell 32:209–216.

Jaenisch R, Breindl M, Harbers K, Jähner D, Löhler J. 1985a. Retroviruses and insertional mutagenesis. Cold Spring Harbor Symp Quant Biol 50:439–445.

Jaenisch R, Schnieke A, Harbers K. 1985b. Treatment of mice with 5-azacytidine efficiently activates silent retroviral genomes in different tissues. Proc Natl Acad Sci USA 82:1451–1455.

Jähner D, Jaenisch R. 1985a. Chromosomal position and specific demethylation in enhancer sequences of germ line-transmitted retroviral genomes during mouse development. Mol Cell Biol 5:2212–2220.

Jähner D, Jaenisch R. 1985b. Retrovirus induced de novo methylation of flanking host sequences correlates with gene inactivity. Nature 315:594–596.

Jähner D, Stuhlmann H, Stewart CL, et al. 1982. De novo methylation and expression of retroviral genomes during mouse embryogenesis. Nature 298:623–628.

Löhler J, Timpl R, Jaenisch R. 1984. Embryonic lethal mutation in mouse collagen I gene causes rupture of blood vessels and is associated with erythropoietic and mesenchymal cell death. Cell 38:597–607.

Müncke M, Harbers K, Jaenisch R, Francke K. 1986. Chromosomal mapping of four different integration sites of Moloney leukemia virus including the locus for αl(I) collagen in mouse. Cytogenet Cell Genet 43:140–149.

Palmiter RD, Brinster R. 1985. Transgenic mice. Cell 41:343–345.

Reik W, Weiher H, Jaenisch R. 1985. Replication-competent Moloney murine leukemia virus carrying a bacterial suppressor tRNA gene: Selective cloning of proviral and flanking host sequences. Proc Natl Acad Sci USA 82:1141–1145.

Schnieke A, Harbers K, Jaenisch R. 1983. Embryonic lethal mutation in mice induced by retrovirus insertion into the alpha 1(I) collagen gene. Nature 304:315–320.

Soriano P, Jaenisch R. 1986. Retroviruses as probes for mammalian development: Allocation of cells to the somatic and germ cell lineages. Cell 46:19–29.

Soriano P, Cone RD, Mulligan RC, Jaenisch R. 1986. Tissue specific and ectopic expression of genes introduced into transgenic mice by retroviruses. Science 234:1409–1413.

Soriano P, Gridley T, Jaenisch R. 1987. Retroviruses and insertional mutagenesis in mice: Proviral integration at the Mov 34 locus leads to early embryonic death. Genes and Development (in press).

Stewart CL, Stuhlmann D, Jäahner D, Jaenisch R. 1982. De novo methylation, expression, and infectivity of retroviral genomes introduced into embryonal carcinoma cells. Proc Natl Acad Sci USA 79:4098–4102.

Stewart C, Harbers K, Jähner D, Jaenisch R. 1983. X chromosome-linked transmission and expression of retroviral genomes microinjected into mouse zygotes. Science 221:760–762.

Stuhlmann H, Jähner D, Jaenisch R. 1981. Infectivity and methylation of retroviral genomes is correlated with expression in the animal. Cell 26:221–232.

Stuhlmann H, Cone R, Mulligan R, Jaenisch R. 1984. Introduction of a selectable gene into different animal tissue by a retrovirus recombinant vector. Proc Natl Acad Sci USA 81:7151–7155.

ONCOGENIC EXPRESSION

Symposium on Fundamental Cancer Research, Vol. 39.
© 1987 by The University of Texas System Cancer Center.

6. Proto-oncogene Expression and Growth Factors during Liver Regeneration

Nelson Fausto, Janet E. Mead, Lundy Braun, Nancy L. Thompson,
Marilyn Panzica, Michele Goyette, Graeme I. Bell,*
and Peter R. Shank[†]

*Department of Pathology and Laboratory Medicine and [†]Section of Molecular,
Cell, and Developmental Biology, Brown University, Providence, Rhode Island 02912
and *Department of Biochemistry and Molecular Biology,
University of Chicago, Chicago, Illinois 60637*

When growth is stimulated in normally quiescent hepatocytes, steady-state levels of c-*fos*, c-*myc*, and p53 mRNAs increase sequentially and transiently before DNA replication. C-*fos* mRNA increases almost immediately after partial hepatectomy and decreases by 2 hr; c-*myc* mRNA reaches maximal levels between 30 min and 2 hr. In contrast, the p53 mRNA increase corresponds to the G_1/S transition, and mRNAs from c-*ras* genes are elevated later, coinciding with DNA replication and mitosis. p53 and p21 proteins are elevated when their mRNAs are more abundant. This regulated response suggests that these genes either control key steps in the cell cycle or are responding to humoral or internal growth factors acting at specified growth stages. We propose that hepatocytes go through a "priming" stage during the first four hours after partial hepatectomy and that their progression through late G_1 is likely to be controlled by autocrine or paracrine mechanisms, which may account for the precisely regulated growth of the liver after partial hepatectomy.

Transforming growth factor beta (TGF β) is a potent inhibitor of DNA synthesis in normal hepatocytes in vitro. We show that TGF β mRNA increases in the regenerating liver at the time of hepatocyte DNA synthesis and mitosis. In normal or regenerating liver, the mRNA for this growth factor is contained in nonparenchymal cells but not in hepatocytes. We suggest that TGF β may be a component of a paracrine regulatory loop that controls hepatocyte replication.

Liver parenchymal cells (hepatocytes) perform a wider range of metabolic functions than any other mammalian cell type. Although hepatocytes of adult animals continuously respond to metabolic signals generated both inside and outside of the liver, these cells rarely divide. In rats, mitosis occurs in only 1 in 20,000 hepatocytes after the first month of life, and many hepatocytes do not replicate throughout the adult life of the animal. However, hepatocytes of adult animals retain the capacity to replicate and readily do so in response to a decrease in cell number caused by cell death or loss of liver tissue (see Bucher and Malt 1971, Wright and Alison 1984 for reviews). The most useful experimental system to study hepatocyte replication has been the regeneration of the liver that takes place after partial hepatectomy, a simple surgical procedure in which 70% of the liver is removed. After partial hepatectomy in rats, the liver remnant grows rapidly; its mass doubles in 24 hr, and after about ten days it weighs as much as the intact liver of a rat of similar age (Higgins and Anderson 1931).

The increase in liver mass after partial hepatectomy, commonly called liver regeneration, is in reality a process of compensatory growth, in which the liver lobes that are removed in the operation do not grow back. Instead, liver mass is restored by the increase in size of the remaining lobes caused by cell replication. As such, liver regeneration shares only a distant relationship with true regenerative processes, such as amphibian limb growth after amputation, where growth originates in a blastema.

A few important characteristics of liver regeneration after partial hepatectomy should be singled out:

1. organ mass is restored by the replication of mature hepatocytes; there is little evidence for "dedifferentiation" of mature cells or replenishment of liver tissue by replication of "stem" cells;

2. the growth process is regulated and does not become autonomous, terminating when organ mass is restored;

3. despite the fact that growth factors, both positive and negative, may be released in the plasma during liver regeneration, the growth response is specific for the liver;

4. the events leading to the first wave of DNA replication are synchronized, making the system suitable for experimental analysis.

During the last few years, we have attempted to determine whether the early events of the regenerative response after partial hepatectomy in rats involve the activation of a large number of genes and, at the same time, to identify genes that may be important as regulators or markers for the prereplicative phase of liver regeneration (Scholla et al. 1980, Fausto et al. 1982, Fausto 1984, Thompson et al. 1986). The results obtained in these studies suggested to us that the prereplicative phase of liver regeneration might be subdivided into stages, each involving different signals and recognized by the expression of specific proto-oncogenes (Fausto and Shank 1986). In this chapter, we review some general features of liver regeneration after partial hepatectomy and present data on proto-oncogene expression and the synthesis of growth factor mRNAs in the regenerating liver.

RNA ACCUMULATION AND OVERALL GENE EXPRESSION DURING THE PREREPLICATIVE PHASE OF LIVER REGENERATION

After partial hepatectomy in rats, DNA synthesis does not increase until 12–15 hr after the operation. It reaches a peak at approximately 24 hr and is followed by a wave of mitosis with a maximum at 30 hr (Grisham 1962). These events represent the synchronized replicative response of hepatocytes, but other liver cells, such as endothelial and Kupffer cells, also proliferate. DNA synthesis in these cells occurs at least 24 hr later than hepatocyte DNA replication. In young rats, a second wave of hepatocyte DNA synthesis occurs (Bucher et al. 1964). After that, the synchronization is lost, but a low level of cell division continues until the mass of the organ is restored in 10–14 days.

The overall rates of RNA synthesis increase by 50%–100% during the first 3–6 hr of regeneration (Fujioka et al. 1963, Bucher and Swafield 1969). The labeling of rRNA is elevated by about fourfold at around 4 hr after partial hepatectomy and remains high at this level for the next 12 hr (Glazer 1977, Walker and Whitfield 1981). It is not known whether these changes reflect increases in transcription, stabilization, or processing of rRNA (Friedman et al. 1984, Powell et al. 1984), but the actual concentration of rRNA per cell is 50% higher than normal 10 hr after partial hepatectomy (Atryzek and Fausto 1979). The kinetics of labeling and accumulation of polyadenylated mRNA in regenerating liver differ from those of rRNA (Fig. 6.1). The concentration of polysomal poly(A)$^+$ RNA/cell (Atryzek and Fausto 1979) increases rapidly (2.5-fold elevation by 12 hr), but the labeling of poly(A)$^+$ HnRNA and polysomal RNA (Glazer 1976, Walker and Whitfield 1981) is elevated only dur-

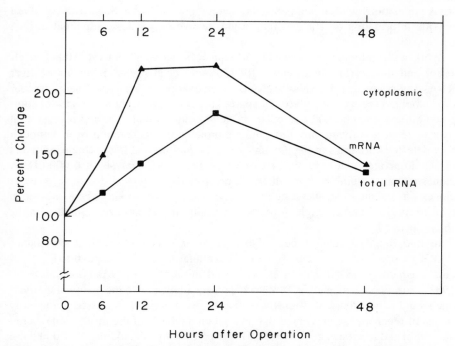

Figure 6.1 Changes in the number of poly(A)$^+$ RNA molecules (▲) and total RNA (■) in rat liver cytoplasm after partial hepatectomy. Poly(A)$^+$ and total RNA concentrations per mg of DNA are given as a percentage of the respective value in unoperated rats (3.35 × 10^{13} cytoplasmic poly(A)$^+$ RNA molecules/mg DNA and 2.29 mg of total cytoplasmic RNA/mg DNA). The abscissa shows the time after partial hepatectomy in hours. (Redrawn from Atryzek and Fausto 1979.)

ing a brief period of time after the operation (twofold increase between 2 and 4 hr after partial hepatectomy, returning to normal by 6 hr). Since HnRNA labeling reflects, at least in part, the transcriptional rate of mRNAs, it is likely that after partial hepatectomy there is only a brief period of time (no more than 2–4 hr) at the start of the process when mRNA synthesis is increased. This conclusion is in keeping with the effect of actinomycin D at early and late stages of the prereplicative period (Gaza et al. 1973, Thompson et al. 1986).

Because of the relatively large increase in mRNA concentration that takes place in the first 12 hr after partial hepatectomy, it was assumed that a very large number of genes became "derepressed" at the early stages of regeneration. The earlier results obtained by nucleic acid hybridization of regenerating liver RNA appeared to confirm these assumptions (Church and McCarthy 1967). However, detailed studies from our and other laboratories (Tedeschi et al. 1978, Wilkes et al. 1979, Grady et al. 1979, Fausto 1984) showed that regeneration involves primarily quantitative rather than qualitative changes in gene expression. In the normal liver, about 6% of the single-copy genome is active, and this proportion appears to change little after partial hepatectomy. Instead, there are changes in the abundance (increases and decreases) of mRNAs that exist in normal liver. These conclusions were reached by analyzing the kinetics and saturation levels of hybridization of regenerating liver RNA populations with homologous and heterologous cDNAs. Such data could not provide information on changes that might involve only a few individual mRNA species.

Work with individual cloned cDNA sequences derived from rat (Huber et al. 1986) and mouse (Friedman et al. 1984, Powell et al. 1984) regenerating liver RNAs has confirmed the view that massive activation of genes or "dedifferentiation" does not seem to take place after partial hepatectomy. Huber et al. (1986) compared 800 soluble and 800 particulate proteins from normal liver and regenerating liver at 18 hr and found only three unique proteins in regenerating liver, although they detected variations in the amounts of individual normal liver proteins in livers of sham-operated and partially hepatectomized rats. An analysis of 6,000 cDNA clones prepared from 18 hr regenerating rat liver RNA showed that none of these clones was unique to regenerating liver. Three clones were found to be expressed at two- to fourfold higher levels in livers of partially hepatectomized rats than in the sham-operated rats.

In BALB/c 3T3 cells stimulated by serum or platelet-derived growth factor (PDGF), approximately 0.2%–0.4% of the cellular mRNA correspond to G_1 "specific" sequences. PDGF causes a 20-fold induction of two RNAs (Cochran et al. 1983, Linzer and Nathans 1983). If such data are applicable to the mammalian liver, one would expect that 20–40 mRNAs may be preferentially expressed at the early stages of regeneration, a number that is high on the basis of the results of Huber et al. (1986) and Friedman et al. (1984). However, even the methodology used in these studies might not be sensitive enough to detect very low abundance mRNAs that might be G_1 specific in hepatocytes.

Changes in the levels of individual mRNAs after partial hepatectomy appear to be in a range of only two- to sixfold. Although further studies may uncover larger numbers of mRNAs that are unique for the prereplicative stage of liver regeneration, it is important to keep in mind that hepatocyte replication in vivo differs significantly from the growth response of cells in culture. Hepatocytes in their physiological stage do not normally divide, but most cells in culture replicate continuously, unless prevented by serum removal or high cell density.

PROTO-ONCOGENE EXPRESSION DURING LIVER REGENERATION

In searching for genes whose expression might change after partial hepatectomy, we found that the abundance of some proto-oncogene mRNAs increases in a transient and sequential manner in regenerating liver (Thompson et al. 1986). This highly regulated pattern of gene expression might offer clues to explain the self-limiting nature of liver regeneration. The proto-oncogene response after partial hepatectomy is not generalized in that c-*src*, c-*abl*, and c-*mos* expression does not change (Fausto and Shank 1983).

The expression of c-Ha-*ras* and c-Ki-*ras* increases by two- to four- and eight- to tenfold, respectively, over that of sham-operated rats and coincides with the major wave of hepatocyte DNA synthesis and mitosis after partial hepatectomy (Goyette et al. 1983). The level of p21 proteins in the liver increases by about twofold between 24 and 72 hr after the operation, but it was not possible to distinguish separately the p21 proteins encoded by the various genes of the c-*ras* family (Thompson et al. 1986). Similar observations on the changes in c-*ras* mRNA abundance during liver regeneration have been reported by various laboratories (Makino et al. 1984b, Corcos et al. 1984). In the regeneration of the liver induced by CCl$_4$ injury, c-Ha-*ras* expression coincides with the wave of DNA synthesis that occurs at about 48 hr after the administration of the chemical (Goyette et al. 1983).

Our earlier work showed that during liver regeneration after partial hepatectomy, the expression of c-*myc* precedes that of c-*ras* (Goyette et al. 1984). Makino et al. (1984a), using a third exon *myc* DNA probe, demonstrated that the abundance of c-*myc* mRNA increases rapidly after partial hepatectomy 1–2 hr after the operation) and that c-*myc* mRNA can be induced by cycloheximide in normal or regenerating liver. Our more recent work, done with the same type of *myc* probe used by Makino et al. (1984a), confirmed their observations and provided a more complete picture of the sequential nature of c-*fos*, c-*myc*, p53, and c-*ras* genes during liver regeneration (Thompson et al. 1986).

We divide the expression of proto-oncogenes after partial hepatectomy into early (0–4 hr), intermediate (8–14 hr), and late (24–72 hr), according to the time of increase of their mRNAs. The c-*fos* and c-*myc* oncogenes belong to the early category: c-*fos* mRNA increases almost immediately after partial hepatectomy, reaches a maximum ½ hr after the operation, and returns to normal by 2 hr (Fig. 6.2). The increase in c-*myc* mRNA is slower, reaching a maximum at 2 hr and returning to normal by 3–4 hr after partial hepatectomy (Fig. 6.2). The expression of the p53 gene falls into the intermediate category. The levels of its mRNA and protein increase 8–16 hr after partial hepatectomy, but the mRNA levels return to normal at

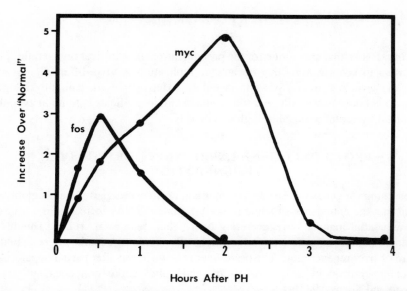

Figure 6.2. C-*fos* and c-*myc* mRNA levels after partial hepatectomy. Total poly(A)$^+$ RNA was prepared from livers of partially hepatectomized rats at the times indicated on the abscissa. Each RNA preparation (5μg) was separated by electrophoresis on a 1.1% formaldehyde/agarose gel, transferred to a nitrocellulose filter and hybridized with ^{32}P-labeled *fos* (1-kb *Pst*I fragment of v-*fos*) or *myc* (*Sal*I-*Pst*I fragment of pv-*myc*) probes. The corresponding bands on the films were quantitated by densitometry. The ordinate indicates the increase in c-*fos* or c-*myc* transcripts in regenerating liver in relationship to values from livers of sham-operated animals. The abscissa shows the time at which partially hepatectomized and sham-operated rats were killed. (Data from Thompson et al. 1986.)

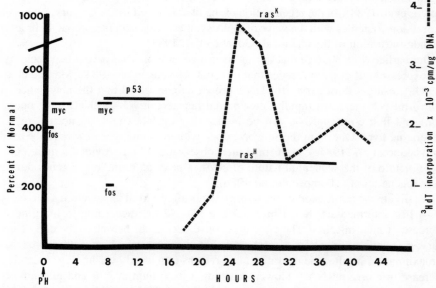

Figure 6.3. Proto-oncogene expression during liver regeneration. Abscissa, times after partial hepatectomy (PH); left ordinate, approximate relative level of expression of various proto-oncogenes in relationship to levels in normal rat liver; horizontal bars, times during liver regeneration at which mRNA levels for each oncogene are elevated; the height of the bars corresponds to peak values which generally occur at the middle of the time period represented; right ordinate, amount of [^{3}H]thymidine incorporation into DNA at various times after PH (_ _ _).

the time of maximal DNA synthesis. Finally, the c-*ras* family genes represent late expression genes, as discussed above (Thompson et al. 1986).

This orderly picture (Fig. 6.3) is confounded somewhat by our finding that there is a second burst of c-*myc* and c-*fos* expression that occurs 8 hr after partial hepatectomy (Thompson et al. 1986). We do not know if the second wave of expression of these two genes represents events taking place in hepatocytes as they progress to DNA synthesis or if it reflects the entry into the cell cycle of liver cells other than hepatocytes that divide later during regeneration. Kruijer et al. (1986) have found that c-*fos* mRNA increases not only in partially hepatectomized rats but is also induced in hepatocytes in culture stimulated by the addition of rat serum, insulin, glucagon, and epidermal growth factor (EGF). In these cultures, the c-*fos* mRNA increase occurred at 30 min after stimulation, while c-*ras* expression occurred 6–24 hr. A biphasic elevation in c-*myc* mRNA was reported by Curran et al. (1985) in NIH 3T3 cells stimulated to proliferate by 20% fetal calf serum. In this case there was a large induction of c-*myc* RNA at 1 hr and a smaller one 6 hr after serum addition.

PROTO-ONCOGENE EXPRESSION AS MARKERS FOR STAGES OF THE PREREPLICATIVE PHASE OF LIVER REGENERATION

The sequential and regulated expression of proto-oncogenes during the prereplicative phase of liver regeneration suggests that the products of these genes have controlling roles in the cell cycle or that they change in abundance as a consquence of events mediated by other signals. In either case, the expression of proto-oncogenes in regenerating liver can serve as useful markers for defining stages in the prereplicative period and for the identification of humoral or cellular stimuli that may act at each of these stages.

For obvious reasons, one of the major themes of research on liver regeneration has been the identification of humoral factors that may trigger the response. Most of these studies, done in vivo or in culture, measure hepatocyte DNA synthesis or replication as an end point. If, however, the regenerative response is a succession of events, each dependent on the preceding stage and with its own set of mediators, it is unlikely that a single factor would be capable of eliciting the full response culminating in DNA synthesis. Instead, it seems logical to subdivide the growth response into stages and to use the expression of specific proto-oncogenes as intermediary end points (Fausto and Shank 1986). It may then be possible to search for mediators that may enhance or modify the expression of these genes at each stage.

The response of hepatocytes after partial hepatectomy involves the interplay between specific effectors (positive or negative) and hepatocyte responsiveness to these effectors. Although quite different from the growth of cells in culture, in analogy to these systems (Pledger et al. 1977), it might be useful to separate the prereplicative phase of liver regeneration into two broad stages (Fig. 6.4). The first stage can be conceived as a "priming" or "competence" phase, representing the transition of hepatocytes from G_0 to G_1. It may last for about 4 hr and is characterized by increased expression of c-*fos* and c-*myc*. The increase in c-*myc* mRNA at

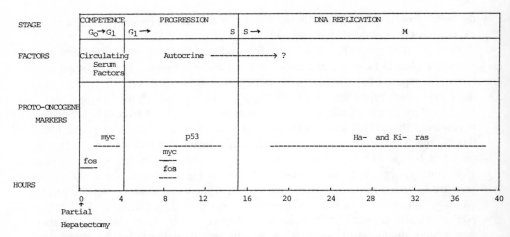

Figure 6.4. Hypothetical scheme of hepatocyte growth stages during liver regeneration.

this stage is entirely blocked by small doses of actinomycin D at the time of the operation (Thompson et al. 1986).

Since the expression of these two genes changes (especially that of c-*fos*) almost immediately after partial hepatectomy, it is likely that mediators for this stage are already present in the blood or are instantaneously released (Cruise et al. 1985). It is also conceivable that c-*fos* and c-*myc* respond to physiological adaptations, such as changes in amino acid (McGowan et al. 1979) and Na^+ (Kruijer et al. 1986) concentrations, which take place in hepatocytes very rapidly after partial hepatectomy. Although such metabolic changes may have no direct relationship to cell replication, they may make nonreplicating hepatocytes capable of responding to growth signals that induce the further steps needed for triggering DNA synthesis. These "primed" hepatocytes then enter a second phase ("progression"), which is characterized by changes in p53 mRNA. Because liver regeneration is a highly controlled and self-limiting growth process, we have suggested that the "progression" stage involves autocrine or paracrine regulatory mechanisms. It is not known whether the initiation of DNA synthesis, which is associated with c-*ras* expression, automatically follows the "progression" stage or if it requires still another set of mediators. Our identification of cell cycle stages in this context is purely arbitrary and is used only as a convenient label (Baserga 1985).

The scheme presented above, although oversimplified (for instance it leaves out the changes in c-*fos* and c-*myc* detected in 8 hr regenerating liver), can be tested experimentally. We have tried to develop systems to demonstrate the "priming" of hepatocytes in intact animals and have also investigated the existence of autocrine or paracrine mechanisms during liver regeneration in vivo.

"PRIMING" OF HEPATOCYTES FOR DNA SYNTHESIS IN VIVO MAY REQUIRE ELEVATED c-myc EXPRESSION

Since hepatocyte proliferation in adult animals occurs as a compensatory response to loss of liver cells or tissue mass, it is difficult to elicit hepatocyte replication in intact normal adult liver. However, it has been known for many years that mouse or rat hepatocytes in the intact animal may respond with a burst of DNA synthesis several hours after the animals are fed high-protein diets (Leduc 1949, Short et al. 1973). This growth response occurs only in animals maintained on protein-free diets for a few days before receiving the protein meal. J. McGowan (Shriners Burn Institute, Boston, Mass.) devised a simple way to induce DNA synthesis in hepatocytes of intact rats (Bucher et al. 1978). The protocol consists of maintaining rats on 20% glucose as the sole source of nutrients and, after three days, giving each of these animals a single dose of amino acids (casein hydrolysate) by stomach tube. The amino acid administration results in a sharp increase in DNA synthesis of approximately 17-fold, which reaches a maximum in 15 hr and declines precipitously by 20 hr (Bucher et al. 1978). Hepatocytes of rats that are starved or normally fed for three days before amino acid administration show no increase in DNA synthesis. As neither starvation nor the glucose regimen cause cell death during the three-day period, the stimulation of DNA synthesis in rats receiving glucose cannot be a result of cell losses. Although the mechanisms involved in the "priming" phenomenon are not known, feeding rats a protein-free diet or a diet deficient only in methionine has the same effect as glucose (Bailey et al. 1976).

Using the conditions described by Bucher et al. (1978), we gave rats 20% glucose as the sole source of food for three days, while a control group was maintained on a normal diet. We extracted RNA from livers of rats receiving glucose or normally fed and measured c-myc mRNA levels (Fig. 6.5). C-myc mRNA was elevated at 24

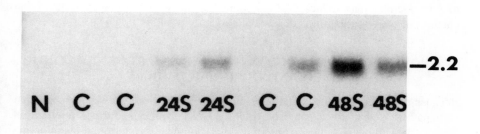

Figure 6.5. C-*myc* mRNA in intact rats normally fed or given 20% glucose as the sole source of food. Groups of rats were normally fed or given 20% glucose as the sole source of food for 1–3 days. Individual rats were killed at 24, 48, 60, and 72 hr after the start of the regimen. Total poly(A) RNA was extracted from individual rats, separated by electrophoresis in formaldehyde/agarose gels and hybridized with ^{32}P-labeled c-*myc* probe (see legend to Fig. 6.1). The figure shows the autoradiographs of RNA preparations from normally fed (C) and sucrose fed (S) individual rats killed at the start of the feeding (N) and 24 and 48 hr later. The 2.2-kb c-*myc* mRNA band is indicated.

hr of glucose feeding and was highest 48 hr after the start of the glucose regimen, although the levels were still higher than normal in animals given glucose for 60 and 72 hr. In contrast, of 10 normally fed animals, which served as controls, only one showed an increase in liver c-*myc* mRNA (Fig. 6.5). These results indicate that c-*myc* mRNA increases in livers of rats in which hepatocytes have been "primed" to undergo DNA synthesis in response to an amino acid load. In contrast, c-*myc* mRNA does not change (with one exception) in rats in which hepatocytes are not capable of DNA replication after amino acid stimulation. It is thus possible that the elevation of c-*myc* mRNA in glucose-fed rats is associated with a "priming" event that makes hepatocytes capable of responding to growth signals not normally recognized by "unprimed" cells.

While the magnitude of DNA synthesis after amino acid loading is comparable in animals maintained for two or three days on 20% glucose, c-*myc* mRNA levels are maximal at two days. We speculate that if c-*myc* expression is related to the "priming" of hepatocytes, this phenomenon is more likely dependent on a secondary event induced by the increase in c-*myc* expression rather than directly related to the actual levels of c-*myc* mRNA. However, we do not know whether the *myc* protein increases and remains elevated at the same time as its mRNA or even if the change in c-*myc* mRNA abundance is the cause or consequence of a "priming" phenomenon. The dietary shift could lead to an elevation of c-*myc* mRNA in the liver by several different mechanisms. One possible explanation is that the glucose regimen, although not causing a decrease in the overall rate of hepatic protein synthesis (Bucher et al. 1978, McGowan et al. 1979), may alter the synthesis or stability of a hypothetical *myc* repressor protein (Makino et al. 1984a).

Maximal DNA synthesis in rats given glucose as the sole source of food for three days takes place at about 15–17 hr after amino acid administration (Bucher et al. 1978, Fausto N., unpublished data). This is considerably earlier (about 7–9 hr) than the peak of DNA synthesis after partial hepatectomy, suggesting that "priming" by glucose feeding may induce G_0-to-G_1 transition in resting hepatocytes involving changes in c-*myc* expression.

GROWTH FACTOR mRNAs IN NORMAL AND REGENERATING LIVER AND IN PURIFIED CELLS

Because of the biologic characteristics of liver regeneration, we hypothesized that in hepatocytes that are capable of entering DNA synthesis, further progression through the cell cycle and cessation of cell division may be controlled by autocrine or paracrine mechanisms (Fausto and Shank 1986). We therefore measured the mRNA levels for two growth factors, transforming growth factor (TGF)-β and insulinlike growth factor (IGF)-II in normal and regenerating liver and undertook cell isolation studies to identify liver cell types that might synthesize these mRNAs. TGF-β mRNA, which is barely detectable in normal liver, increases in livers of rats at about 4 hr after partial hepatectomy. These levels do not change further until about 18 hr after the operation, when they increase again, reach a maximum at 72 hr, and return to approximately normal levels by 96 hr (Fausto N., unpublished

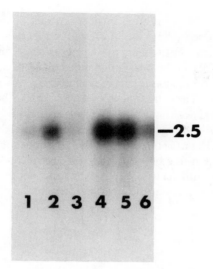

Figure 6.6. TGF-β mRNA during liver regeneration. Polysomal poly(A) $^+$ mRNA from partially hepatectomized rats was separated by electrophoresis and hybridized with [^{32}P]TGF-β probe (1.1-kb Bgl 1 fragment from human TGF-β cDNA clone 2 prepared by G. I. Bell, Univ. of Chicago). Lane 1, normal rat; lanes 3 and 6, sham-operated rats at 4 and 48 hr after operation respectively; lanes 2, 4, and 5, partially hepatectomized rats at 4, 24, and 48 hr after operation. The line indicates the 2.5-kb TGF-β mRNA.

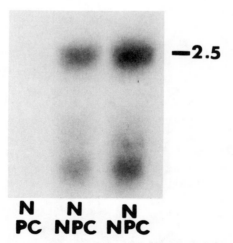

Figure 6.7. TGF-β mRNA in different liver cell types. Whole cell RNA obtained from normal liver hepatocytes (PC) and nonparenchymal (NPC) cells was hybridized with TGF-β cDNA probe. The line indicates the 2.5-kb TGF-β mRNA.

data). TGF-β mRNA did not change in livers of rats killed 2–96 hr after sham operation. Some of these findings are illustrated in Figure 6.6.

Although hepatocytes constitute approximately 90% of the total liver mass, they represent only about 65% of the total cell population. If the accumulation of TGF-β mRNA during liver regeneration is part of an autocrine growth control mechanism, this mRNA must be present in hepatocytes and should thus be detectable in hepatocytes purified from regenerating livers. We isolated hepatocytes and nonparenchymal cells from normal and regenerating livers using methods previously described (Yaswen et al. 1984, Hayner et al. 1984). The techniques involve the perfusion of the livers with a calcium-free buffer followed by perfusion with collagenase. This two-step procedure is sufficient for hepatocyte isolation. However, to purify nonparenchymal cells, it is necessary to treat the collagenase-dissociated tissue (freed

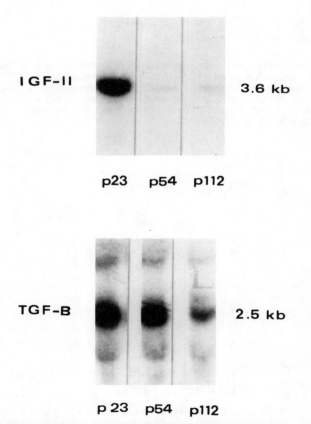

Figure 6.8. Expression of TGF-β and IGF-II mRNAs in liver epithelial cells in culture. Liver epithelial cells (oval cells) were obtained by centrifugal elutriation from livers of rats fed a carcinogenic diet (choline deficient containing .05% DL-ethionine) for six weeks (Yaswen et al. 1984, Braun et al. 1986). Whole cell RNA was obtained from cultures at various passages as indicated on the figure and hybridized with human TGF-β or IGF-II cDNA probes (Bell et al. 1984). The 3.6-kb and 2.5-kb bands corresponding to IGF-II and TGF-β mRNAs, respectively, are indicated.

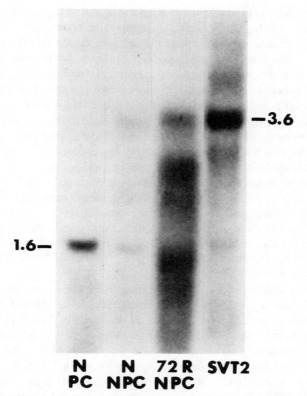

Figure 6.9. IGF-II mRNA in different liver cell types. Hybridization of IGF-II [^{32}P]cDNA probe with whole cell RNA from normal hepatocytes (N-PC) and nonparenchymal cells from normal liver (N-NPC) and 72 hr regenerating liver (72R-NPC). RNA obtained from SVT2 cell line is shown to indicate the position of the 3.6-kb IGF II mRNA. Note that nonparenchymal cells from normal liver contain a faint 3.6-kb band while normal hepatocytes contain a strong 1.6-kb band.

of most hepatocytes) with a mixture containing collagenase, pronase, and DNase, which digests the remaining hepatocytes and the connective tissue framework while preserving nonparenchymal cells. We isolated RNAs from hepatocytes and nonparenchymal cells purified from normal and regenerating livers and hybridized them with TGF-β cDNA. Much to our surprise, we detected the 2.5-kb TGF-β mRNA band in RNA from normal liver nonparenchymal cells but not in normal liver hepatocyte preparations (Fig. 6.7). Similarly, we detected the 2.5-kb TGF-β mRNA band in nonparenchymal cells purified from regenerating liver at 24, 48, and 72 hr but not in RNA preparations from hepatocytes purified from these same livers (Fausto N., unpublished data). Our results, so far, have led us to conclude that the synthesis of TGF-β increases during liver regeneration in rats and that nonparenchymal cells might be the source for this growth factor in the liver. Hepatocytes from normal or regenerating liver seem to contain only very low levels of TGF-β mRNA or none at all.

The nonparenchymal cell fractions we have analyzed so far are heterogeneous and include epithelial cells, Kupffer cells, and endothelial cells. Purification of discrete cell types will be necessary to pinpoint the cell type responsible for TGF-β mRNA synthesis in normal and regenerating rat liver. However, we have found that TGF-β mRNA also increases during liver carcinogenesis in rats receiving a carcinogenic diet (choline deficient, containing 0.05% ethionine) at a time when liver epithelial cells (oval cells) proliferate (Fausto N., unpublished data). We have purified these epithelial cells by centrifugal elutriation, characterized the cells, and placed them in culture (Fausto et al. 1986). The elutriated epithelial cell fraction contains approximately 10% Kupffer cells (peroxidase staining) and appears to be free of endothelial cells. The liver epithelial cells in culture produce large amounts of TGF-β and IGF-II mRNAs, up to about passage 60 for TGF-β and passage 30 for IGF-II (Fig. 6.8). At these stages, the cells do not grow in soft agar, are not tumorigenic in nude mice, and show regulated expression of proto-oncogenes during the cell cycle. At later passages, the synthesis of TGF-β mRNA decreases considerably, and IGF-II transcripts become undetectable altogether. At these later stages, the cells are still nontumorigenic but have acquired the capacity to grow in soft agar in the presence of EGF (Braun et al. 1987).

Our studies of IGF-II mRNA in regenerating liver have so far failed to reveal any consistent changes in this mRNA during regeneration. The situation is complicated by the existence of multiple IGF-II RNAs, as described by Soares et al. (1985) and Graham et al. (1986). The 3.6-kb IGF-II mRNA band is very abundant in fetal liver but decreases drastically in newborn rats (Fausto N., unpublished data). In cells purified from normal adult livers, hepatocytes do not contain 3.6-kb IGF-II mRNA but have instead a smaller IGF-II of approximately 1.6 kb. However, we detected the 3.6-kb IGF-II mRNA in nonparenchymal cells from normal and regenerating livers (Fig. 6.9) and, in large amounts, in liver epithelial cells in culture (Fig. 6.8).

A WORKING HYPOTHESIS: TWO-STAGE MODEL OF LIVER REGENERATION

Our work, although still at a very early stage, suggests that changes in c-*myc* mRNA in hepatocytes of intact adult rats (nonpartially hepatectomized) may be associated with a "priming" event that makes these nonreplicating cells capable of undergoing DNA synthesis upon amino acid stimulation. Although triggered by different mediators, a similar priming event may occur in hepatocytes during the first hours after partial hepatectomy. It is possible that at this stage of regeneration, hepatocytes become able to respond to or synthesize growth effectors, which may induce further progression through the cell cycle.

We also show here that TGF-β mRNA increases during liver regeneration at about the time of the wave of hepatocyte DNA synthesis and mitosis. However, both TGF-β and IGF-II mRNAs appear to be produced in the liver by nonparenchymal cells rather than hepatocytes. At least one nonparenchymal cell type, that is, liver epithelial cells, synthesize large amounts of these mRNAs at early passages in culture. These results raise some interesting questions and suggest a number of alternative interpretations. It is possible that the synthesis of TGF-β and IGF-II mRNA by nonparenchymal cells and the increase in TGF-β mRNA after partial hepatectomy are unrelated to hepatocyte DNA synthesis and replication. Another interpretation is that the synthesis of growth factor mRNAs by nonparenchymal cells might be part of paracrine growth mechanisms that regulate liver regeneration. If one assumes that the synthesis of TGF-β and IGF-II mRNAs by liver nonparenchymal cells is in some way related to hepatocyte replication, a further complication arises in that TGF-β has been reported to inhibit EGF-stimulated hepatocyte DNA synthesis (Nakamura 1985, Carr et al. 1986, McMahon et al. 1986) in culture. However, TGF-β is a bifunctional factor (Roberts et al. 1985, Goustin et al. 1986) that stimulates or inhibits growth of the same cell type depending on the physiological state of the cells and the interaction with other growth factors. Moreover, in the only situation so far where TGF-β effects in vivo have been studied in detail, that is, wound healing in rats, TGF-β had stimulatory effects (Roberts and Sporn 1985). Thus, it is possible that TGF-β is a positive effector for hepatocytes in vivo and that it would have similar effects on "primed" hepatocytes in culture.

If further experiments prove that TGF-β functions as an inhibitor of hepatocyte DNA synthesis in vivo, it is necessary to explain why the synthesis of a growth inhibitor increases during a growth process. The paradox might be more apparent than real because proliferation-inhibitory factors may be needed in feedback mechanisms required for regulated growth and differentiation (Masui et al. 1986, McMahon et al. 1986). It is thus possible that the increase in TGF-β synthesis in the liver after partial hepatectomy may prevent the uncontrolled proliferation of hepatocytes during liver regeneration. It is conceivable that TGF-β inhibits DNA replication in quiescent hepatocytes in normal liver and in newly divided hepatocytes in the regenerating liver but does not block DNA synthesis in "primed" hepatocytes at the prereplicative phase of liver regeneration. A similar mechanism for regulated growth control may occur in lymphocytes. TGF-β mRNA increases almost 10-fold in stimulated lymphocytes (Derynck et al. 1985), although this growth factor inhibits IL-2–dependent T lymphocyte proliferation (Kehrl et al. 1986). Similarly, the induction of an interferonlike gene by PDGF in BALB/c 3T3 cells (Zullo et al. 1985) is another example of the synthesis of a growth inhibitory substance triggered by cell growth.

The possibility that liver regeneration involves a "priming" stage followed by paracrine regulatory mechanisms is a novel but untested idea. If a two-stage sequence exists in vivo, the "priming" event must lead to changes in hepatocyte responsiveness to growth factors rather than to their synthesis by hepatocytes. The effectors involved may also include those synthesized outside the liver, such as EGF (Earp and O'Keefe 1981). Indeed, it has been shown that in culture EGF stimulates DNA synthesis in hepatocytes from regenerating liver to a greater extent than normal liver hepatocytes (Richman et al. 1976, Francavilla et al. 1986). Further work may show that hepatocytes not only respond to but also synthesize many different growth factors and that the interaction between these factors and receptor availability regulates the regenerative response. In any event, the hypotheses discussed in this paper can be validated or discarded by further experiments.

ACKNOWLEDGMENT

This investigation was supported by grants CA 23226 and CA 35249 awarded by the National Cancer Institute, United States Department of Health and Human Services. We thank Ms. Anna-Louise Baxter for help in preparing the manuscript and Michael McGuire for his excellent work.

REFERENCES

Atryzek V, Fausto N. 1979. Accumulation of polyadenylated mRNA during liver regeneration. Biochemistry 18:1281–1287.

Bailey RP, Vrooman MJ, Sawai Y, Tsukada K, Short J, Lieberman I. 1976. Amino acids and control of nucleolar size, the activity of RNA polymerase I, and DNA synthesis in liver. Proc Natl Acad Sci USA 73:3201–3205.

Baserga R. 1985. The Biology of Cell Reproduction. Harvard University Press, Cambridge, MA, pp. 134–210.

Bell GI, Merryweather JP, Sanchez-Pescador R, et al. 1984. Sequence of a cDNA clone encoding human preproinsulin-like growth factor II. Nature 310:775–777.

Braun L, Goyette M, Yaswen P, Thompson NL, Fausto N. 1987. Liver epithelial cells from carcinogen-treated rats: Growth in culture and tumorigenicity after transfection with the *ras* oncogene. Cancer Res (in press).

Bucher NLR, Malt RA. 1971. Regeneration of Liver and Kidney. Little, Brown and Co., Boston, pp. 17–176.

Bucher NLR, Swaffield MN. 1969. Ribonucleic acid synthesis in relation to precursor pools in regenerating rat liver. Biochim Biophys Acta 174:491–502.

Bucher NLR McGowan JA, Patel U. 1978. Hormonal regulation of liver growth. ICN-UCLA Symposia on Molecular and Cellular Biology. 12:661–670.

Bucher NLR, Swaffield MN, DiTroia JF. 1964. Influence of age upon incorporation of thymidine-2-C^{14} into DNA of regenerating rat liver. Cancer Res 24:509–512.

Carr BI, Hayashi I, Branum EL, Moses HL. 1986. Inhibition of DNA synthesis in rat hepatocytes by platelet-derived type β transforming growth factor. Cancer Res 46:2330–2334.

Church RB, McCarthy BJ. 1967. Ribonucleic acid synthesis in regenerating and embryonic liver. I. The synthesis of new species of RNA during regeneration of mouse liver after partial hepatectomy. J Mol Biol 23:459–476.

Cochran BH, Reffel AC, Stiles CD. 1983. Molecular cloning of gene sequences regulated by platelet-derived growth factor. Cell 33:939–947.

Corcos D, Defer N, Ramondjean M. et al. 1984. Correlated increase of the expression of the c-*ras* genes in chemically induced hepatocarcinomas. Biochem Biophys Res Commun 122:259–264.

Cruise JL, Houck K, Michalopoulos GK. 1985. Induction of DNA synthesis in cultured rat hepatocytes through stimulation of α adrenoreceptor by norepinephrine. Science 277:749–751.

Curran T, Bravo R, Muller R. 1985. Transient induction of c-fos and c-myc is an immediate consequence of growth factor stimulation. Cancer Surveys 4:655–681.

Derynck R, Jarrett JA, Chen EY, et al. 1985. Human transforming growth factor-β complementary DNA sequence and expression in normal and transformed cells. Nature 316:701–705.

Earp HS, O'Keefe EJ. 1981. Epidermal growth factor receptor number decreases during rat liver regeneration. J Clin Invest 67:1580–1583.

Fausto N. 1984. Messenger RNA in regenerating liver: implications for the understanding of regulated growth. Mol Cell Biochem 59:131–147.

Fausto N, Shank PR. 1983. Oncogene expression in liver regeneration and carcinogenesis. Hepatology 3:1016–1023.

Fausto N, Shank PR. 1986. Analysis of proto-oncogene expression during liver regeneration and hepatic carcinogenesis. *In* Okuda K, Ishak KG, eds., Neoplasms of the Liver. Springer-Verlag, New York.

Fausto N, Schultz-Ellison G, Atryzek V, Goyette M. 1982. Distribution and specificity of sequences in polyadenylated nuclear RNA of normal, regenerating and neoplastic liver. J Biol Chem 257:2200–2206.

Fausto N, Thompson NL, Braun L. 1986. Purification and culture of oval cells from rat liver. *In* Pretlow TP, Pretlow TG, eds., Cell Separation: Methods and Selected Applications, vol. 4, Academic Press, Orlando, pp. 45–77.

Francavilla A, Ove P, Polimeno L, Sciascia C, Coetzee ML, Starzl TE. 1986. Epidermal growth factor and proliferation in rat hepatocytes in primary culture isolated at different times after partial hepatectomy. Cancer Res 46:1318–1323.

Friedman JM, Chung EY, Darnell JE Jr. 1984. Gene expression during liver regeneration. J Mol Biol 179:37–53.

Fujioka M, Koga M, Lieberman I. 1963. Metabolism of ribonucleic acid after partial hepatectomy. J Biol Chem 238:3401–3406.

Gaza DJ, Short J, Lieberman I. 1973. Transcriptional and translational control of the biphasic increase in ornithine decarboxylase activity in liver. Biochem Biophys Res Commun 54:1483–1488.

Glazer RI. 1976. The action of cordycepin on nascent nuclear RNA and poly(A) synthesis in regenerating liver. Biochim Biophys Acta 418:160–166.

Glazer RI. 1977. The action of N-hydroxy-2-acetylaminofluorene on the synthesis of ribosomal and poly(A)-RNA in normal and regenerating liver. Biochim Biophys Acta 475:492–500.

Goustin AS, Leof EB, Shipley GD, Moses HL. 1986. Growth factors and cancer. Cancer Res 46:1015–1029.

Goyette M, Petropoulos CJ, Shank PR, Fausto N. 1983. Expression of a cellular oncogene during liver regeneration. Science 219:510–512.

Goyette M, Petropoulos CJ, Shank PR, Fausto N. 1984. Regulated transcription of c-ki-*ras* and c-*myc* during compensatory growth of rat liver. Mol Cell Biol 4:1493–1498.

Grady LJ, Campbell WP, North AB. 1979. Nonrepetitive DNA transcription in normal and regenerating rat liver. Nucleic Acids Res 7:259–269.

Graham DE, Rechler MM, Brown AL, et al. 1986. Coordinate developmental regulation of high and low molecular weight mRNAs for rat insulin-like growth factor II. Proc Natl Acad Sci USA 83:4519–4523.

Grisham JW. 1962. Morphologic study of deoxyribonucleic acid synthesis and cell proliferation in regenerating rat liver: Autoradiography with thymidine-H^3. Cancer Res 22:842–849.

Hayner NT, Braun L, Yaswen P, Brooks M, Fausto N. 1984. Isozyme profiles of oval cells, parenchymal cells and biliary cells isolated by centrifugal elutriation from normal and preneoplastic livers. Cancer Res 44:332–338.

Higgins GM, Anderson RM. 1931. Experimental pathology of liver. I. Restoration of liver of white rat following partial surgical removal. Arch Pathol 12:186–202.

Huber BE, Heilman CA, Wirth PJ, Miller MJ, Thorgeirsson SS. 1986. Studies of gene transcription and translation in regenerating rat liver. Hepatology 6:209–219.

Kehrl JH, Wakefield LM, Roberts AB, et al. 1986. Production of transforming growth factor β by human T lymphocytes and its potential role in the regulation of T cell growth. J Exp Med 163:1037–1050.

Kruijer W, Skelly H, Botteri F, et al. 1986. Proto-oncogene expression in regenerating liver is simulated in cultures of primary adult rat hepatocytes. J Biol Chem 261:7929:7933.

Leduc EH. 1949. Mitotic activity in the liver of the mouse during inanition followed by refeeding with different levels of protein. Am J Anat 84:397–421.

Linzer DIH, Nathans D. 1983. Growth-related changes in specific mRNAs of cultured mouse cells. Proc Natl Acad Sci USA 80:4271–4275.

Makino R, Hayashi K, Sugimura T. 1984a. C-*myc* transcript is induced in rat liver at very early stage of regeneration or by cycloheximide treatment. Nature 310:697–698.

Makino R, Hayashi K, Sato S, Sugimura T. 1984b. Expression of the c-Ha-*ras* and c-*myc* genes in rat liver tumors. Biochem Biophys Res Commun 119:1096–1102.

Masui T, Wakefield LM, Lechner JF, La Veck MA, Sporn MB, Harris CC. 1986. Type β transforming growth factor is the primary differentiation-inducing serum factor for normal human bronchial epithelial cells. Proc Natl Acad Sci USA 83:2438–2442.

McGowan J, Atryzek V, Fausto N. 1979. Effects of protein deprivation on the regeneration of rat liver after partial hepatectomy. Biochem J 180:25–35.

McMahon JB, Richards WL, delCampo AA, Song M-KH, Thorgeirsson SS. 1986. Differential effects of transforming growth factor-β on proliferation of normal and malignant rat liver epithelial cells in culture. Cancer Res 46:4665–4671.

Nakamura T, Tomita Y, Hirai R, Yamaoka K, Kaji K, Ichihara A. 1985. Inhibitory effect of transforming growth factor-β on DNA synthesis of adult rat hepatocytes in primary culture. Biochem Biophys Res Commun 133:1042–1050.

Pledger WJ, Stiles CD, Antoniades HN, Sher CD. 1977. Induction of DNA synthesis in BALB/c3T3 cells by serum components: Reevaluation of the commitment process. Proc Natl Acad Sci USA 74:4481–4485.

Powell DJ, Friedman JM, Oulette AJ, Krauter KS, Darnell JE Jr, 1984. Transcriptional and post-transcriptional control of specific messenger RNAs in adult and embryonic liver. J Mol Biol 179:21–35.

Richman RA, Claus TH, Pilkis SJ, Friedman DL. 1976. Hormonal stimulation of DNA synthesis in primary cultures of adult rat hepatocytes. Proc Natl Acad Sci USA 73:3589–3593.

Roberts AB, Sporn MB. 1985. Transforming growth factors. Cancer Surveys 4:683–705.

Roberts AB, Anzano MA, Wakefield LM, Roche NS, Stern DF, Sporn MB. 1985. Type beta transforming growth factor: a bi-functional regulator of cellular growth. Proc Natl Acad Sci USA 82:119–123.

Scholla C, Tedeschi MV, Fausto N. 1980. Gene expression and the diversity of polysomal messenger RNA sequences in regenerating liver. J Biol Chem 225:2855–2860.

Soares MB, Ishii DN, Efstratiadis A. 1985. Developmental and tissue-specific expression of a family of transcripts related to rat insulin-like growth factor II mRNA. Nucleic Acids Res 13:1119–1134.

Short J, Armstrong NB, Zemel R, Lieberman I. 1973. A role for amino acids in the induction of deoxyribonucelic acid synthesis in liver. Biochem Biophys Res Commun 50:430–437.

Tedeschi MV, Colbert DA, Fausto N. 1978. Transcription of the non-repetitive genome in liver hypertrophy and the homology between nuclear RNA of normal and 12h-regenerating liver. Biochim Biophys Acta 521:641–649.

Thompson NL, Mead JE, Braun L, Goyette M, Shank PR, Fausto N. 1986. Sequential protooncogene expression during rat liver regeneration. Cancer Res 46:3111–3117.

Walker PR, Whitfield JF. 1981. Regulation of the prereplicative changes in the synthesis and transport of messenger and ribosomal RNA in regenerating livers of normal and hypocalcemic rats. J Cell Physiol 108:427–437.

Wilkes PR, Birnie GD, Paul J. 1979. Changes in nuclear and polysomal polyadenylated RNA sequences during rat liver regeneration. Nucleic Acids Res 6:2193–2208.

Wright N, Alison M. 1984. The Biology of Epithelial Cell Populations. Clarendon Press, Oxford, pp. 880–980.

Yaswen P, Hayner NT, Fausto N. 1984. Isolation of oval cells by centrifugal elutriation and comparison with other cell types purified from normal and preneoplastic livers. Cancer Res 44:324–331.

Zullo J, Cochran BH, Huang AS, Stiles CD. 1985. Platelet-derived growth factor and double-stranded ribonucleic acids stimulate expression of the same genes in 3T3 cells. Cell 43:793–800.

Symposium on Fundamental Cancer Research, Vol. 39.
© 1987 by the University of Texas System Cancer Center.

7. The *Drosophila* Epidermal Growth Factor Receptor Homolog: Structure, Evolution, and Possible Functions

Ben-Zion Shilo, Eyal D. Schejter, Daniel Segal, *Dorit S. Ginsberg, and Lillian Glazer

*Departments of Virology and *Neurobiology,
The Weizmann Institute of Science, Rehovot 76100, Israel*

A unique gene termed DER (*Drosophila* epidermal growth factor [EGF] receptor homolog) was isolated from *Drosophila melanogaster* and mapped to position 57F on the right arm of the second chromosome. The deduced amino acid sequence showed that the DER protein is 1409 amino acids long. In homology it is similar to the human EGF receptor and to rat and human *neu* proteins. The most striking difference between the *Drosophila* and human homologs is DER's additional 166 amino acids. The extra sequence is rich in cysteine residues and is another duplication of one of the two cysteine-rich regions, which are a hallmark of the EGF receptor and related proteins.

Analysis of several cDNA clones of DER revealed variability at the 5' end of the coding region, demonstrating the presence of at least three splicing alternatives. All three transcripts have a similar tissue distribution during development: they are uniformly distributed in embryos, localized primarily in proliferating tissues in larvae, and found mainly in the brain cortex and the thoracic and abdominal ganglia in adults. The DER protein thus seems to have multiple roles during development, and it may represent a "universal" transducer of signals into the cell.

Membrane receptors represent a crucial component in the transduction of signals from the external environment into the cell. Several receptors have been implicated in the transmission of mitogenic stimuli. Initially, this prediction was based on the observations that growth-stimulating factors such as insulin, epidermal growth factor (EGF), platelet-derived growth factor (PDGF), or insulinlike growth factor I bind to specific receptors at the cell surface. Moreover, binding of these factors to their respective receptors stimulated an intrinsic tyrosine kinase activity of the receptors, suggesting that the different receptors have structural similarities and may belong to a common gene family (Kasuga et al. 1982, Ushiro and Cohen 1980, Ek et al. 1982, Jacobs et al. 1983).

The involvement of membrane receptors in normal processes of growth control became more evident from the findings that several oncogenes represent modified versions of growth factors or their receptors. Initially, the v-*sis* oncogene was shown to be derived from the gene coding for the β chain of PDGF (Waterfield et al. 1983, Doolittle et al. 1983). Subsequently the v-*erb*B oncogene was shown to be a truncated version of the EGF receptor (Downward et al. 1984b), and the *neu* oncogene derived from a rat glio/neuroblastoma turned out to be structurally similar to the EGF receptor (Schechter et al. 1984). The list of oncogenes representing membrane receptors is growing and includes also the v-*fms* oncogene, derived from the colony-stimulating factor 1 (CSF-1) receptor (Sherr et al. 1985), the v-*ros* oncogene (being highly similar but not identical to the insulin receptor) (Ullrich et al. 1985, Ebina et al. 1985), and possibly the *mas* oncogene, which may represent a totally new type of oncogene resembling the β adrenergic receptor and the rhodopsins (Young et al., 1986).

The EGF, *neu*, insulin, and CSF-1 receptors have two major features in common. All have a single hydrophobic transmembrane domain and a cytoplasmic tyrosine kinase domain (Ullrich et al. 1984, 1985, Bargmann et al. 1986a, Yamamoto et al. 1986, Coussens et al. 1986, Ebina et al. 1985, Hampe et al. 1984). These receptors differ in their ligand-binding specificities, and the structure of the extracellular domains varies accordingly. This report will concentrate on a *Drosophila* gene that is homologous to the genes coding for both EGF and *neu* receptors. We will, therefore, review briefly the available data on these vertebrate receptors and raise some of the questions that remain open.

Based on the nucleotide sequence of cDNA clones (Ullrich et al. 1984), the EGF receptor contains four distinct domains: an N-terminal EGF–binding domain, a transmembrane segment, a kinase domain, and a C-terminal region that probably has regulatory functions. It is synthesized as a 134-kDa precursor from which the N-terminal signal peptide is cleaved to generate a 131-kDa polypeptide. The molecule is then N-glycosylated to yield the mature 170-kDa protein. The external EGF-binding domain is a cysteine-rich sequence of 621 amino acids. The transmembrane segment contains only 23 amino acids and presumably traverses the membrane only once. Immediately internal to the membrane is a short basic region and a threonine residue that is phosphorylated by kinase C (Hunter et al. 1984). The following region is homologous in structure to the tyrosine kinase domain of several oncogenes and is followed by a C-terminal fragment that can be cleaved from the receptor. This fragment contains the three major sites of tyrosine autophosphorylation (Downward et al. 1984a).

The *neu* oncogene was initially identified by transfection into NIH 3T3 cells of DNA extracted from a rat glio/neuroblastoma induced by transplacental introduction of ethylnitrosourea (Shih et al. 1981). Isolation of the rat and human *neu* genes has shown that they are very similar in sequence and overall organization to the EGF receptor. The structure of the two human receptors is summarized in Figure 7.1. In spite of the significant sequence homology between the extracellular domains of the EGF and *neu* receptors (41%), the two molecules are apparently not activated by the same ligand. While the tyrosine kinase activity of the EGF receptor was shown to be stimulated by EGF and α-TGF (Cohen et al. 1980, Todaro et al. 1980), these ligands, as well as a wide spectrum of other ligands, do not enhance the tyrosine

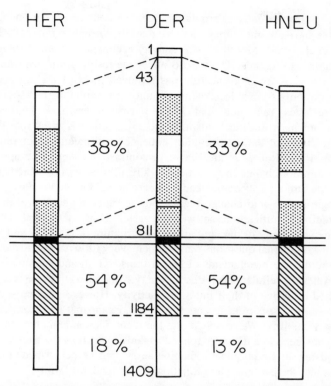

Figure 7.1. Alignment of the putative DER protein with the EGF receptor (HER) and human *neu* (HNEU). The kinase domains are shown by hatched boxes, the transmembrane domain by black boxes, and the cystene-rich domains by dotted boxes. The percentage of homology is shown.

kinase activity of the *neu* protein (Stern et al. 1986); thus the ligand that triggers it remains unknown.

One of the striking features of the extracellular sequence of the EGF and *neu* receptors is the presence of cysteine-rich domains of about 170 residues, each containing 20–24 cysteines. Both receptors contain two such domains, which may result from a duplication of a single cysteine-rich domain. A single cysteine domain has also been found in the α chain of the insulin receptor. The wide distribution of cysteine-rich domains suggests that they play a crucial role in the function of receptors. Their function may be associated with the aggregation or internalization of receptors rather than with actual binding of ligands, since receptors with different binding specificities share the same domains. Also, the local disulphide bonds that are likely to form within these domains may generate a structure that is too rigid for ligand binding.

One intriguing question is by what mechanism does ligand binding at the extracellular domain of the receptor trigger kinase activity in the cytoplasmic domain. Analysis of the structural alterations leading to oncogenic activation of the EGF and *neu* receptors is instrumental in providing clues. In both cases, the oncogenic protein appears to have a higher kinase activity than its normal counterpart (Kris et al. 1985, Stern et al. 1986). Moreover, this activity is constitutive and does not depend on the availability of ligands. The v-*erb*B oncogene results from two truncations of the EGF receptor. A major truncation has removed most of the extracellular sequence, leaving only 65 residues, while a minor truncation at the C-terminus has removed 32 residues (Yamamoto et al. 1983). In cases of erythroleukemias resulting from a promoter insertion mechanism of the avian leukosis virus into the c-*erb*B gene, the truncation of the extracellular sequence is sufficient to activate the gene (Nilsen et al. 1985, Raines et al. 1985). In contrast, the *neu* gene appears to be activated by a minor change in its structure, a result that was expected, in view of the fact that the tumor has been induced by a carcinogen known to cause point mutations. A single amino acid change (valine 664 to glutamic acid) within the transmembrane region is sufficient to activate the protein (Bargmann et al. 1986b).

Despite the wide body of data regarding the structure of the EGF and *neu* receptors, the major functional questions remain open. Very little is known about the sites of ligand binding, the mechanisms of signal transduction and activation of the kinase, or the relevant cellular substrates for the tyrosine kinase. These receptors have been identified by virtue of their mitogenic activity. However, the prospect of their involvement in processes of differentiation at the organismal level remains an open and exciting possibility. We reasoned that the identification and characterization of the homologous gene in a distantly related organism, such as the fruit fly *Drosophila melanogaster,* in which genetic manipulations can be performed, may provide new insights into the evolution and function of this receptor family.

THE *DROSOPHILA* EGF RECEPTOR HOMOLOG (DER)

Structure

Using sequences containing the kinase domain of v-*erb*B as hybridization probes, a unique homologous gene termed DER was isolated from *Drosophila melanogaster* DNA. Sequence analysis of genomic DER clones demonstrated the presence of a predicted transmembrane domain and extensive homology to the human EGF receptor (HER) in the kinase and extracellular domains (Livneh et al. 1985, Wadsworth et al. 1985). The putative *Drosophila* protein is thus likely to function as a ligand-triggered kinase. The entire cytoplasmic domain of the DER gene is contained within a single exon, and so its amino acid sequence could be deduced from the genomic clone. However, the presence of several introns in the extracellular coding region had prevented unambiguous sequence determination of this domain.

To isolate cDNA clones of the DER gene, we have screened a 3–12 hr embryonic cDNA library using sequences prepared from the genomic region coding for the extracellular domain as hybridization probes. The comparison of DER genomic and cDNA clones demonstrated the presence of four introns within the gene.

The complete structure of the protein can be deduced from the compiled genomic and cDNA sequence (Schejter et al. 1986) and is shown schematically in Figure 7.1. DER encodes a putative protein of 1409 amino acids. It has a signal peptide of 42 residues followed by an extracellular domain of 769 amino acids. A single hy-drophobic transmembrane domain precedes the kinase region and the additional C-terminal domain.

Homology of the DER Protein to the HER and *neu* Receptors

In its overall structure and organization, the DER protein resembles both the EGF and *neu* receptors. Although the DER gene was isolated by a probe prepared from the kinase domain of v-*erb*B (the avian EGF receptor counterpart), it appears to be equally homologous to *neu*. The highest degree of homology is within the kinase domain (54%). Beyond the kinase region the C-terminal domain shows a limited degree of homology among all three proteins. Alignment of the extracellular do-mains again shows a similar degree of homology between the DER and the EGF or *neu* receptors (37% and 33%, respectively). Since the EGF and *neu* receptors are activated by different ligands, it is likely that the common sequences in the ligand-binding domain do not determine the binding specificities. Similarly, because the *Drosophila* receptor is equally homologous to both human receptors, we predict that the ligand that triggers it should be distant from the human ligands. Nevertheless, the *Drosophila* ligand may belong to the EGF/α-TGF family.

A *Drosophila* gene coding for the insulin receptor homolog has recently been iso-lated. In contrast to the DER product, the protein encoded by the *Drosophila* insulin receptor homolog showed elevated kinase activity following addition of insulin (Pe-trozzelli et al. 1986).

Evolution of the EGF Receptor Gene Family

The most striking difference between the *Drosophila* and human receptors is an in-sertion of 166 amino acids in the DER between the second cysteine-rich domain and the transmembrane region. This insertion is also rich in cysteines (20 residues). The known cysteine-rich domains are structurally similar in the spacing of cysteines and in the conservation of several residues between them. It was thus possible to align the additional sequence in the DER protein and show that it is a bona fide cysteine-rich domain (Schejter et al. 1986).

The ability to compare the sequence of the cysteine domains of related receptors in different species provides new insights into the evolution of this receptor family. Alignment of the eight cysteine domains from the DER, HER, *neu*, and insulin re-ceptor proteins shows that they are generally colinear (we will refer to the latter two human receptors as HNEU and HIR, respectively). This pattern is markedly dis-rupted only in two positions. The second cysteine domain of HER and HNEU, as well as the rudimentary extracellular sequence of the avian v-*erb*B, contain an in-sertion of 9–10 amino acids that is absent from all other sequences. Interestingly, the same domains of HER and HNEU also contain an additional, smaller insertion of four amino acids in another position. The presence of these two insertions only in the second domain of HER and HNEU, as well as the additional duplication of a cysteine domain in DER, provide clues to the events that may have shaped the struc-ture of this receptor gene family in the course of evolution.

Since many of the genes from the tyrosine kinase family in diverse species do not contain an extracellular domain, we speculate that the EGF-insulin receptor family was initiated by fusion between a sequence coding for a cytoplasmic tyrosine kinase and a sequence coding for an extracellular region with a single cysteine-rich domain. Similar types of fusions may have occurred multiple times in evolution. Another receptor, the CSF-1 receptor, c-*fms,* shares a tyrosine kinase domain but does not have a cysteine-rich domain within its extracellular portion (Hampe et al. 1984). Following the suggested fusion of the two domains, gene duplication events have generated multiple receptors that provided the precursors of the insulin, EGF, and *neu* receptors, as well as other receptors with tyrosine kinase activity. The specific ancestor of the EGF receptor family has subsequently undergone a duplication of the single cysteine-rich domain.

The dynamic events described so far must have occurred prior to the chordate-arthropod divergence, over 800 million years ago. Following the divergence, the ancestor gene has undergone different sets of changes in the two phyla. In arthropods, an additional duplication of a cysteine domain has occurred, while in chordates, two minor changes in the second cysteine domain have probably generated the 10 and 4 amino acid insertions. Only after the occurrence of these changes has the gene been duplicated in vertebrates to give rise to the EGF receptor and *neu* receptor genes. A model for the evolution of the family is shown in Figure 7.2.

The HER and *neu* genes in vertebrates represent highly similar members of the

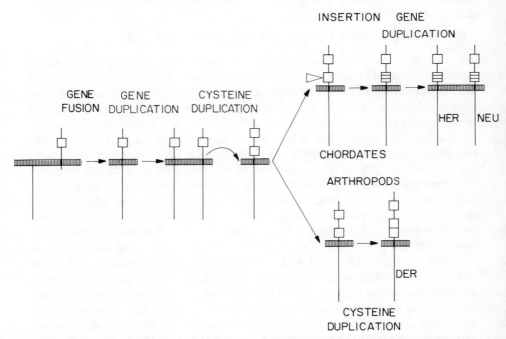

Figure 7.2. A model for the evolution of the EGF receptor gene family. Cysteine-rich domains are shown by boxes.

same family, whereas the DER appears to be a unique gene in *Drosophila*. This is the only gene that was isolated by using the avian v-*erb*B kinase probe (Livneh et al. 1985). In addition, no related genes could be cloned from a *Drosophila* library by using the DER extracellular coding sequence as a probe. Thus, in contrast to vertebrates, a single receptor of this family appears to be sufficient in *Drosophila*.

Alternative 5' Exons of DER Transcripts

Analysis of additional cDNA clones of the DER indicates that this gene generates transcripts coding for three different proteins. Six cDNA clones that span the 5' ends of the gene were isolated from the embryonic 3–12 hr cDNA library. Structural characterization and sequencing of these clones revealed three different structures at the 5' end, which can be attributed to the alternative utilization of 5' exons (Schejter et al. 1986). The effect of this splicing pattern on the structure of the protein is interesting, since each of the three types of transcripts codes for a putative receptor that varies at its N-terminal sequence. In one case, the 5' exon codes only for a signal peptide, whereas in the second case, the exon codes for a signal peptide followed by 70 additional residues. For the third case, only a single cDNA clone was isolated, which codes for 120 amino acids upstream of the point of sequence divergence. However, since this clone is a truncated one, we do not know the full coding capacity of its 5' exons.

What could be the functional implication of the alternative N-terminal structures? The occurrence of this diversity in the extracellular region suggests that it may be involved in ligand binding. It could even be possible that a single receptor gene codes for three or more proteins that would recognize the same ligand with different affinities. Alternatively, each form may respond to a different ligand but would subsequently activate the same common kinase domain. In the absence of information about the ligands in *Drosophila* that trigger the DER protein, these predictions cannot be tested.

Speculation about the Ligands that Trigger the DER

A possible clue to the ligands that may interact with the DER protein has recently emerged from the study of the neurogenic loci of *Drosophila*. Null mutations in seven different loci cause an embryonic-lethal phenotype involving abnormal growth of the embryonic neuroblasts at the expense of ventral ectoderm cells (Lehmann et al. 1983). All of these loci are believed to be involved in the same developmental pathway. The surprising observation was that two of these genes, Notch and Delta, contain 36 and 2 EGF-like repeats, respectively (Wharton et al. 1985, Campos-Ortega J., personal communication, 1986). These findings raise the possibility that the cell's choice between two alternative developmental routes, namely neuroblasts versus ventral ectoderm cells, is made by a process mediated by EGF-like ligands through cell-cell interactions. In the absence of one component in this signal transduction pathway, most cells in the ventral region of the embryos develop into neuroblasts. The presence of EGF-like putative ligands in *Drosophila* and the finding that more than one such ligand participates in the same pathway raise the attractive possibility that the DER protein may be the receptor for Notch and Delta. This notion is currently being tested by genetic and anatomic assays.

Localization of DER Transcripts during Development

The ability to localize transcripts of the DER gene in situ during development has offered some clues as to the function of the gene product (Schejter et al. 1986). Two major conclusions were obtained from these studies. Probes that are specific to each of the 5' exons showed a similar spatial and temporal distribution pattern, which indicates that the three transcripts are made simultaneously in the same tissues. In addition, the transcript distribution pattern suggests that the protein has a dual function during development because it is associated with both cell proliferation at the larval stage and differentiated functions of nondividing tissues in the adult. In embryos, the distribution of transcripts is uniform. The pattern changes dramatically at the larval stage. Those larval tissues, which comprise polytenized, nondividing cells (such as the salivary glands or fat cells), do not express the DER. Localized expression is observed, however, in all dividing diploid tissues, including the imaginal discs (eye-antenna, wing, genital, etc.), the anlagen of the testes and ovaries, and in the brain cortex. In adults, DER transcripts are localized to several tissues, such as the cortex of the brain and the thoracic and abdominal ganglia. The DER protein thus appears to be a general transducer of signals that may trigger different responses in different cell types.

Genetic Approaches

The alternative splicing pattern and the localization of DER transcripts indicate that the protein may have pleiotropic functions during development. These functions can be better understood in the future by utilization of genetic approaches. Such approaches would allow us to carry out, in the context of the whole organism, in vivo studies of experimentally manipulated or mutated versions of the gene. The localization of the DER gene to position 57F on the right arm of the second chromosome (Livneh et al. 1985) has allowed us to obtain regional chromosomal deletions that are currently being used for the isolation of recessive mutants lacking a functional DER gene.

A promising genetic approach is to induce mutant phenotypes corresponding to gain or loss of function mutations of the DER by introduction of additional copies of the DER gene into the germ line via P elements (Spradling and Rubin 1982, Rubin and Spradling 1982). As some of these constructs are expected to have lethal effects, they are placed under the control of the heat shock hsp70 promoter. In one construct, the DER cDNA clone was truncated similarly to the v-*erb*B oncogene, a modification that may render the activity of the kinase domain constitutive. In another construct, an attempt was made to block the normal pathway of DER by expression of high levels of a modified DER gene that codes for an intact extracellular and transmembrane domain but has lost the cytoplasmic kinase region. Such a protein is expected to titrate the normal ligands without transducing the proper signals into the cells.

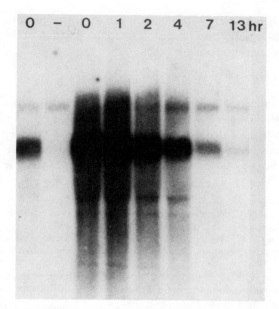

Figure 7.3 Induction of DER expression following heat shock. The DER construct truncated similar to *erb*B was placed under hsp70 promoter in a P element rosy vector. Transformed lines were obtained following embryo injections Adult flies from the transformed line were grown at 24°C and used for RNA extraction either after a 45-minute incubation at 34°C (left lane), without heat shock (next lane), or after a 45-minute incubation at 36.5°C and extraction of RNA at the times indicated following heat shock. 20 μg of total RNA (about one fly equivalent) were loaded on each lane and hybridized with the antisense SP6 probe of DER.

Figure 7.3 shows the induction of DER transcripts by heat shock in flies transformed with the v-*erb*B–like construct of DER. It is clear that the uninduced level is not detectable, while the induced level is two or three orders of magnitude higher than that of the endogenous transcript, which is longer. Furthermore, extraction of RNA from flies at different times after heat shock shows that the induced transcript persists for over seven hours. It should thus be possible to divide the developmental cycle of *Drosophila* into 7–10 hr periods, to induce the expression of the constructs, and monitor the phenotypic effects at each interval. Any phenotypes that are observed should provide a selection system for dominant suppressor mutations in genes coding for proteins that interact with DER. To date, the cellular pathways activated by the family of tyrosine kinases are not known.

CONCLUDING REMARKS

The initial analysis of the putative DER protein structure and the tissue localization of transcripts point to two levels of complexity. First, DER transcripts code for at least three types of proteins. Second, the gene is expressed in different tissue types during development, including both proliferating and differentiated cells. Genetic analysis should help to clarify the pleiotropic roles of the putative receptor during development. These roles may be analogous to the function of the vertebrate EGF and *neu* receptors during morphogenesis.

ACKNOWLEDGMENT

This work was supported by grants from the U.S.-Israel Binational Fund and the Julia and Leo Forchheimer Foundation for Molecular Genetics to Ben-Zion Shilo, who is an incumbent of the Hass Career Development Chair, and by grants from the Israel Academy of Sciences Basic Research Fund and the Israel Cancer Research Fund to Daniel Segal, who is an incumbent of the Charles Clore fellowship.

REFERENCES

Bargmann CI, Hung M-C, Weinberg RA. 1986a. The *neu* oncogene encodes an epidermal growth factor receptor–related protein. Nature 319:226–230.

Bargmann CI, Hung M-C, Weinberg RA. 1986b. Multiple independent activation of the *neu* oncogene by a point mutation altering the transmembrane domain of p185. Cell 45: 649–657.

Cohen S, Carpenter G, King L Jr. 1980. Epidermal growth factor-receptor–protein kinase interactions: Co-purification of receptor and epidermal growth factor–enhanced phosphorylation activity. J Biol Chem 255:4834–4842.

Coussens L, Yang-Feng TL, Kiao Y-C, et al. 1986. Tyrosine kinase receptor with extensive homology to EGF receptor shares chromosomal location with *neu* oncogene. Science 230:1132–1139.

Doolittle RF, Hunkapiller MW, Hood LE, et al. 1983. Simian sarcoma virus onc gene v-*sis* is derived from the gene (or genes) encoding a platelet derived growth factor. Science 221: 275–277.

Downward J, Parker, P, Waterfield MD. 1984a. Autophosphorylation sites on the epidermal growth factor receptor. Nature 311:483–485.

Downward J, Yarden Y, Mayes E, et al. 1984b. Close similarity of epidermal growth factor receptor and v-*erb*B oncogene protein sequences. Nature 307:521–527.

Ebina Y, Ellis L, Jarnagin K, et al. 1985. The human insulin receptor cDNA: The structural basis for hormone-activated transmembrane signalling. Cell 40:747–758.

Ek B, Westermark B, Westerson A, Heldin CH. 1982. Stimulation of tyrosine-specific phosphorylation by platelet-derived growth factor. Nature 295:419–420.

Hampe A, Gobet M, Sherr CJ, Galibert F. 1984. Nucleotide sequence of the feline retroviral oncogene v-*fms* shows unexpected homology with oncogenes encoding tyrosine-specific protein kinases. Proc Natl Acad Sci USA 81:85–89.

Hunter T, Ling N, Cooper JA. 1984. Protein kinase C phosphorylation of the EGF receptor at a threonine residue close to the cytoplasmic face of the plasma membrane. Nature 311: 480–483.

Jacobs S, Kull FC Jr, Earp HS, Svoboda ME, Van Wyk JJ, Cuatrecasas P. 1983. Somatomedin-C stimulates the phosphorylation of the subunit of its own receptor. J Biol Chem 258:9581–9584.

Kasuga M, Zick Y, Blithe DL, Crettaz M, Kahn CR. 1982. Insulin stimulates tyrosine phosphorylation of the insulin receptor in a cell-free system. Nature 298:667–669.

Kris RM, Lax I, Gullick W, et al. 1985. Antibodies against a synthetic peptide as a probe for kinase activity of the avian EGF receptor and v-*erb*B protein. Cell 40:619–625.

Lehmann R, Jiminez F, Dietrich U, Campos-Ortega J. 1983. On the phenotype and development of mutants of early neurogenesis in *Drosophila melanogaster*. Roux's Archives of Developmental Biology 192:62–79.

Livneh E, Glazer L, Segal D, Schlessinger J, Shilo B-Z. 1985. The *Drosophila* EGF receptor homolog: Conservation of both hormone binding and kinase domains. Cell 40:599–607.

Nilsen TW, Maroney PA, Goodwin RG, et al. 1985. c-*erb*B activation in ALV-induced erythroblastosis: Novel RNA processing and promoter insertion result in expression of an amino-truncated EGF receptor. Cell 41:719–726.

Petruzzelli L, Herrera R, Arenas-Garcia R, Fernandez R, Birnbaum M, Rosen OM. 1986. Isolation of a *Drosophila* genomic sequence homologous to the kinase domain of the human insulin receptor and detection of the phosphorylated *Drosophila* receptor with an anti-peptide antibody. Proc Natl Acad Sci USA 83:4710–4714.

Raines MA, Lewis WG, Crittenden LB, Kung H-J. 1985. c-*erb*B activation in avian leukosis virus-induced erythroblastosis: Clustered integration sites and the rearrangement of provirus in the c-*erb*B alleles. Proc Natl Acad Sci USA 82:2287–2291.

Rubin GM, Spradling AC. 1982. Genetic transformation of *Drosophila* with transposable element vectors. Science 218:348–353.

Schechter AL, Stern DF, Vaidyananthan L, et al. 1984. The *neu* oncogene. An *erb*B related gene encoding a 185,000-Mr tumour antigen. Nature 312:513–516.

Schejter ED, Segal D, Glazer L, Shilo B-Z. 1986. Alternative 5' exons and tissue-specific expression of the *Drosophila* EGF receptor homolog transcripts. Cell 46:1091–1101.

Sherr CJ, Rettenmier CW, Sacca R, Roussel MF, Look AT, Stanely ER. 1985. The c-*fms* proto-oncogene product is related to the receptor for the mononuclear phagocyte growth factor, CSF-1. Cell 41:665–676.

Shih C, Padhy LC, Murray M, Weinberg RA. 1981. Transforming genes of carcinomas and neuroblastomas induced into mouse fibroblasts. Nature 290:261–264.

Spradling AC, Rubin GM. 1982. Transposition of cloned P elements into *Drosophila* germ line chromosomes. Science 218:341–347.

Stern DF, Hefferman PA, Weinberg RA. 1986. p185, a product of the *neu* proto-oncogene, is a receptor-like protein associated with tyrosine kinase activity. Mol Cell Biol 6:1729–1740.

Todaro GJ, Fryling C, De Larco JE. 1980. Transforming growth factors produced by certain human tumor cells: Polypeptides that interact with epidermal growth factor receptors. Proc Natl Acad Sci USA 77:4258–5261.

Ullrich A, Coussens L, Hayflick JS, et al. 1984. Human epidermal growth factor receptor cDNA sequence and aberrant expression of the amplified gene in A431 epidermoid carcinoma cells. Nature 309:418–425.

Ullrich A, Bell JR, Chen EY, et al. 1985. Human insulin receptor and its relation to the tyrosine kinase family of oncogenes. Nature 313:756–761.

Ushiro H, Cohen S. 1980. Identification of phosphotyrosine as a product of epidermal growth factor–activated protein kinase in A431 cell membranes. J Biol Chem 255:8363–8365.

Wadsworth SC, Vincent WS, Bilodeau-Wentworth D. 1985. A *Drosophila* genomic sequence with homology to human epidermal growth factor receptor. Nature 314:178–180.

Waterfield MD, Scarce GT, Whittle N, et al. 1983. Platelet-derived growth factor is structurally related to the putative transforming protein p28[sis] of simian sarcoma virus. Nature 304:35–39.

Wharton KA, Johnson KM, Xu T, Artavanis-Tsakonas S. 1985. Nucleotide sequence from the neurogenic locus Notch implies a gene product that shares homology with proteins containing EGF-like repeats. Cell 43:567–581.

Yamamoto T, Nishida T, Miyajima N, Kawai S, Oui T, Toyoshima K. 1983. The *erb*B gene of avian erythroblastosis virus is a member of the *src* gene family. Cell 35:71–78.

Yamamoto T, Ikawa S, Akiyama T, et al. 1986. Similarity of protein encoded by the human *erb*B-2 gene to epidermal growth factor receptor. Nature 319:230–234.

Young D, Waitches G, Birchmeier C, Fasano O, Wigler M. 1986. Isolation and characterization of a new cellular oncogene encoding a protein with multiple potential transmembrane domains. Cell 45:711–719.

Symposium on Fundamental Cancer Research, Vol. 39.

8. Proto-oncogene *fos:* An Inducible Multifaceted Gene

Richard L. Mitchell, Steven K. Hanks, and Inder M. Verma

The Salk Institute, San Diego, California 92138

Proto-oncogene *fos*, which is expressed during cell growth and cell differentiation and development, is a multifaceted gene. The viral homolog, v-*fos*, was identified as the resident transforming gene of FBJ-murine osteosarcoma virus, which induces bone tumors in mice. Owing to an in-frame deletion during the biogenesis of the v-*fos* gene, the products of viral and cellular *fos* proteins differ at their C-termini. Despite different C-termini, both *fos* proteins are nuclear in their location and can transform fibroblasts in vitro. However, transformation by the c-*fos* gene requires removal of a 67-base pair sequence from the 3′ noncoding domain. Proto-oncogene *fos* is a highly inducible gene in response to a variety of growth factors and differentiation-specific inducers. The expression of the *fos* gene is not modulated during the cell cycle.

The realization that normal cells harbor genes that have the potential of inducing neoplasia has been a turning point in modern cancer research. Such genes are commonly called proto-oncogenes (c-*onc*) because they are the progenitors of the viral oncogenes (v-*onc*) that were first discovered in transforming retroviruses (Bishop 1983, 1985a, Hunter 1984). DNA transfection techniques have facilitated the isolation of additional transforming genes not found in retroviruses. To date, nearly three dozen oncogenes have been identified and the list is growing (Cooper 1982, Weinberg 1983, Bishop 1985b). It thus seems paradoxical that the cell remains normal in the face of such potential adversity. Why has the cell not lost these potentially lethal genes during the course of evolution?

As we ascertain the functions of oncogenes, their preservation during evolution becomes more understandable. To cite an example, the proto-oncogene *fms* protein is likely the receptor for macrophage colony-stimulating factor and hence pivotal in the generation of mature macrophages (Sherr et al. 1985). Similarly, proto-oncogene *sis* encodes the β-chain of platelet-derived growth factor (PDGF), a potent mitogen involved in connective tissue repair and wound healing (Doolittle et al. 1983, Waterfield et al. 1983, Ross et al. 1986). What events conspire to convert these essential cellular genes to acquiring transforming potential? We have used proto-oncogene *fos* as a model system to understand the precarious balance between essential cellular functions and cellular transformation.

BACKGROUND

Anatomy of the *fos* Gene

Oncogene v-*fos* is the transforming gene of both FBJ- and FBR-murine osteosarcoma viruses (FBJ-MSV, FBR-MSV), which induce bone tumors in vivo and transform fibroblasts in vitro (Finkel et al. 1966, 1972, Curran and Teich 1982, Curran et al. 1982). Mouse and human cells seem to have only a single copy of the cellular progenitor of the v-*fos* gene (Curran et al. 1982). The complete nucleotide sequence of the FBJ- and FBR-MSV proviral DNA and of the mouse and human proto-oncogenes *fos* have been reported (Van Beveren et al. 1983, van Straaten et al. 1983). The salient features may be briefly described as follows (Fig. 8.1):

FBJ-MSV

1. FBJ-MSV proviral DNA contains 4,026 base pairs, including two long terminal repeats (LTR) of 617 base pairs each, 1,639 base pairs of acquired cellular sequence (v-*fos*), and a portion of the viral envelope (*env*) gene.

2. Both the initiation and termination codons of the v-*fos* protein are within the acquired sequences that encode a protein of 381 amino acids, having a molecular weight of 49,601.

3. In cells transformed by FBJ-MSV, a phosphoprotein with an apparent M_r of 55,000 (p55) on sodium dodecyl sulfate polyacrylamide gel electrophoresis (SDS-PAGE) has been identified as the transforming protein (Curran et al. 1982). The discrepancy between the observed size and the size predicted by sequence analysis is probably the result of the unusual amino acid composition of the *fos* protein (10% proline), since the v-*fos* protein expressed in bacteria has a similar mobility on SDS-PAGE (MacConnell and Verma 1983, Verma et al. 1984).

FBR-MSV

1. The proviral DNA of FBR-MSV contains 3,791 base pairs (specifying a genome of 3,284 bases) and encodes a single *gag-fos* fusion product of 554 amino acids (Curran and Verma 1984, Van Beveren et al. 1984).

2. The *fos* portion of the gene lacks sequences that encode the first 24 and the last 98 amino acids of the 380 amino acid mouse c-*fos* gene product. In addition, the coding region has sustained three small in-frame deletions, one in the p30^{gag} portion and two in the *fos* region.

3. The gene product terminates in a sequence termed *fox*, which is present in normal mouse DNA at a locus unrelated to the c-*fos* gene. The c-*fox* gene or genes are expressed as an abundant class of poly(A) RNA in mouse tissue (Van Beveren et al. 1984).

Proto-oncogene fos

1. The sequences in the c-*fos* gene that are homologous to those in the v-*fos* gene are interrupted by four regions of nonhomology, three of which are bona fide introns.

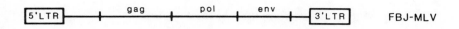

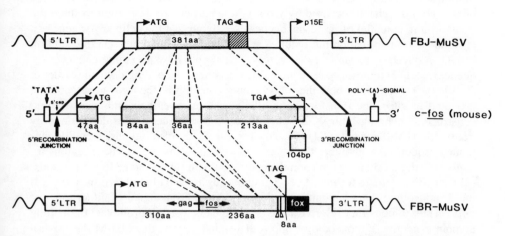

Figure 8.1. Structure of the c-*fos* (mouse) gene and FBJ- and FBR-MSV proviral DNAs. (Top and bottom) 5′ and 3′ long terminal repeats (LTR) sequences of FBJ- and FBR-MSV are depicted by open boxes, other noncoding regions are indicated by a solid line. The portions of the v-*fos* and gag-*fos* genes encoding the viral homologues to c-*fos* are indicated by stippled boxes. (Middle) Exons are depicted by stippled boxes, introns and 5′ and 3′ untranslated regions are indicated by a solid line. Indicated below each exon is the length (in amino acids) of the segment of *fos* protein it encodes. Also indicated in the figure are the TGA termination codon used by c-*fos*, the TAG termination codon used by v-*fos*, and the location of the TATA box, 5′-cap, and poly(A)-addition signal. The data in this figure were compiled from Van Beveren et al. 1983, 1984.

2. The fourth nonhomologous region is present in both mouse and human c-*fos* genes and results from the deletion of 104 base pairs of the cellular sequence.

3. The c-*fos* gene is highly conserved between mouse and human genomes, encoding a protein of 380 amino acids, nearly identical in size to the 381 amino acid v-*fos* protein. Starting at the amino-terminal end, v-*fos* and mouse c-*fos* proteins are nearly identical, differing at only 5 of the first 332 amino acid residues. At this point, the two sequences diverge entirely, and the remaining 49 amino acids at the carboxyl terminus of v-*fos* are completely different from the corresponding 48 residues in c-*fos*. This deletion shifts the translational reading frame and allows the v-*fos* coding sequence to terminate at a TAG codon downstream of the TGA termination codon normally used by the c-*fos* gene.

4. Despite their different carboxyl termini, both the v-*fos* and c-*fos* proteins are located in the nucleus.

5. The c-*fos* protein undergoes more extensive posttranslational modification than the v-*fos* protein.

6. The mouse and human c-*fos* genes share greater than 90% sequence homology, differing at only 24 residues of a total of 380 (Curran et al. 1984).

Transformation by fos Proteins

Both FBJ-MSV and FBR-MSV containing the *fos* gene can transform established fibroblast cell lines (Curran et al. 1982, Curran and Verma 1984). Because human tumors are not generally caused by viruses, it is particularly important to study the transforming potential of proto-oncogenes. We found that the cellular *fos* gene can also induce transformation but requires at least two manipulations: (1) the addition of LTR sequences, presumably to increase transcription by providing enhancer sequences, and (2) removal of sequences downstream of the coding domain (Miller et al. 1984). To determine how the transforming potential of the c-*fos* gene could be activated in vitro, the transformation efficiencies of several recombinant plasmid constructs containing both v-*fos* and mouse c-*fos* sequences were determined by transfection (Miller et al. 1984). The constructs were divided into three regions containing sequences from either the v-*fos* or c-*fos* genes (Fig. 8.2). These regions included (1) the promoter region and the coding domain for the first 316 amino acids, (2) the coding domain for the 64 or 65 amino acids at the carboxyl terminus, and (3) the 3' noncoding domain containing the poly(A) addition signal of either v-*fos* or c-*fos*. Thus, a construct referred to as VVV means that the promoter, the coding domain, and the 3' noncoding region all originate from the FBJ-MSV proviral DNA, while MMM signifies that the complete sequence was derived from the c-*fos*

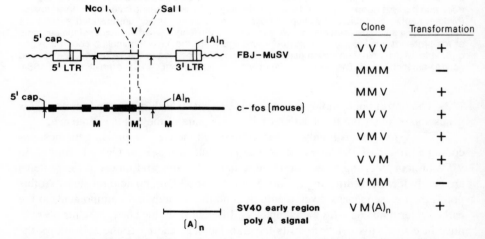

Figure 8.2. Transforming potential of the c-*fos* gene. The top line depicts the FBJ-MSV provirus. The v-*fos* coding region is indicated by an open box in the middle of the provirus. Wavy lines surrounding the provirus indicate cellular flanking sequences. The bottom line depicts the mouse c-*fos* gene with the c-*fos* coding region shown by filled boxes. The coding regions of each of the c-*fos* genes are separated by three introns. The restriction endonucleases *Nco*I and *Sal*I divide the v-*fos* and mouse c-*fos* genes into three regions as shown. RNA 5'-cap and polyadenylation signals are also shown. The origins of these chimeric plasmids have been described (Miller et al. 1984). The arrows below the c-*fos* genome indicate the positions of recombination between the mouse gene and the helper retrovirus that generated FBJ-MSV. Clones were tested for transforming ability by transfection onto rat 208F cells. (+) indicates transformation efficiency of about 200 foci/μg of DNA, (−) indicates transforming efficiency of less than 10 foci/μg of DNA.

mouse gene. The results of these experiments indicate that both v-*fos* and c-*fos* proteins are capable of inducing cellular transformation, but that in order to activate the c-*fos* transforming potential, an active promoter is required and the 3' c-*fos* noncoding domain must be separated from the 3' coding domain.

Construct VMM, which does not induce transformation efficiently, is transcribed but is unable to synthesize sufficient p55^{fos} protein (Miller et al. 1984). In comparison, when the 3' noncoding sequences are removed as in the transforming construct VM(A)$_n$, at least ten times more *fos* protein is synthesized (F. Meijlink and T. Curran, unpublished data). The region of the 3' noncoding domain involved in this interaction has been localized to an AT-rich 67-base pair region located about 500 base pairs downstream from the end of the coding domain and about 120 base pairs upstream of the poly(A) addition signal (Meijlink et al. 1985). Two possible mechanisms may explain the influence of the 67-base pair region: (1) c-*fos* protein synthesis may be regulated by interaction of the 67-base pair region with the c-*fos* protein, or (2) the presence of the 67-base pair region may influence the stability of the c-*fos* mRNA. Sequences including the 67-base pair region have been shown to influence the transient accumulation of transcripts from constructs containing c-*fos* sequences (Treisman 1985).

METHODS

Cell Lines and Culture Conditions

The human promonocytic leukemia cell line U-937 (Sundstrom and Nilsson 1976) was maintained in RPMI-1640 medium supplemented with 10% fetal bovine serum (FBS), penicillin (100 units/ml), streptomycin (100 μg/ml; GIBCO, Grand Island, NY), 2 mM L-glutamine, 0.12% (w/v) NaHCO$_3$, and 2 mM pyruvic acid. Cultures were maintained by passage at a density of 2×10^5 cells/ml every three to five days. For serum starvation, U-937 cells were passaged at a density of 2×10^5 cells/ml in RPMI supplemented with 0.5% FBS and allowed to grow for seven days before serum stimulation by the addition of fresh FBS to a final concentration of 10% (v/v). A fresh solution of each chemical inducer was prepared for each experiment from stock solutions of 1-oleoyl-2-acetyl-*rac*-glycerol (diacylglycerol, or DAG; Sigma Chemical Co., St. Louis, MO; 100 mg/ml in dimethyl sulfoxide, DMSO) or the calcium ionophore A23187 (Sigma; 10 mg/ml in DMSO).

HeLa cells and rat 208F cells were maintained as monolayer cultures grown in Dulbecco's modified Eagle's medium (DMEM) supplemented with 10% FBS and the usual concentrations of antibiotics.

S-Phase Arrest by Double Thymidine Block

HeLa cells were blocked in S phase by the addition of thymidine or aphidicolin. To block cells with thymidine, 3×10^6 HeLa cells were seeded on 150-mm tissue culture plates in 20 ml of DMEM and grown overnight before addition of fresh medium containing 2 mM thymidine. After 24 hr of growth in thymidine, the cultures were rinsed with fresh DMEM, then cultured 12 hr in DMEM lacking thymidine. Cells were then blocked a second time by the addition of fresh DMEM containing 2 mM thymidine. After an additional 12 hr in culture, cells were rinsed with fresh DMEM, then cultured in fresh DMEM until RNA was harvested at the times indicated in the figures to follow. Within 15 min after release of the second thymidine block, more than 95% of the cells were in S phase as determined by flow cytometry.

S-Phase Arrest by Aphidicolin Block

To block cells with aphidicolin, cells were blocked first with a single treatment of thymidine as indicated above, then washed and grown in DMEM lacking thymidine for 12 hr, and then cultured an additional 12 hr in medium containing 5 μg/ml aphidicolin. Cells were released from the block and RNA was harvested as indicated above.

Mitotic Arrest by High-Pressure Nitrous Oxide

Cells were first cultured and blocked with a single treatment with thymidine as described above, and then grown in DMEM lacking thymidine for 3.5 hr and synchronized during mitosis by growth at 37°C in an atmosphere of nitrous oxide at a pressure of 80 pounds per square inch as described previously (Rao 1968). After 8 hr of culture in nitrous oxide, cells were returned to an atmosphere of 95% air, 5% CO_2, and RNA was harvested.

Analysis of Cell Cycle State

Cell cycle state was determined at time intervals after release of cells from S-phase block by flow cytometry as described previously (Gray and Coffino 1979). In brief, cells were harvested by trypsinization, and 10^6 cells were washed twice in trypsin/EDTA. After resuspension in 0.1 ml of residual buffer, 4 ml of cold, filtered 70% ethanol was added dropwise with continuous mixing on a vortex machine. After a 10-min incubation at 4°C, the cells were pelletized and resuspended in 0.5 ml of a solution containing propidium iodide (40 μg/ml) and RNase (40 μg/ml) and then incubated 30 min at 37°C before flow cytometry.

Isolation and Analysis of Total Cellular RNA

Total cellular RNA was isolated by the method of Chirgwin et al. (1979) and analyzed by electrophoresis of 10-μg samples of total RNA through 1.2% agarose formaldehyde gels (Lehrach et al. 1977) followed by transfer to nitrocellulose (Thomas 1980) and hybridization to radiolabeled *fos* or histone H2B probes. Preparations of *fos* probe, histone H2B probe, and hybridization were as previously described (Mitchell et al. 1985, Meinkoth and Wahl 1984, Rigby et al. 1977).

RESULTS

Induction of the *fos* Gene

Expression of the *fos* gene was first observed in mouse extra-embryonal tissue, with the highest levels of expression recorded in day 18 amnion cells (Muller et al. 1982, Muller and Verma 1984). Gonda and Metcalf (1984) reported the identification of *fos* mRNA transcripts during differentiation of monomyelocytic cells. It soon became evident that the c-*fos* gene is highly inducible in response to a variety of agents. Furthermore, the induction is transient. In the past few years c-*fos* gene expression has been observed in a wide variety of cell types in response to a large number of mitogens and differentiation-specific agents.

Several investigators have extensively analyzed the expression of the c-*fos* gene in differentiating monomyelocytes, PC12 cells, and fibroblasts in transit from the G_0 to the G_1 stage of the cell cycle (Gonda and Metcalf 1984, Muller et al. 1984a,b, Mitchell et al. 1985, 1986, Greenberg and Ziff 1984, Kruijer et al. 1984, 1985, Morgan and Curran 1986, Greenberg et al. 1985). Several generalizations can be made:

1. Induction of *fos* is very rapid and generally transient, except in the case of differentiating monocytes or monomyelocytes. Here sustained expression of *fos* is observed at a level that is four- to fivefold lower than the highest levels (Mitchell et al. 1985).

2. c-*fos* Transcripts can be detected within 1 to 2 min of the addition of an inducer, the highest levels accumulating within 30 to 60 min to a maximum of 5 to 10 copies per cell. Within 120 min, c-*fos* transcripts decline to undetectable levels.

3. Addition of the protein synthesis inhibitors cycloheximide or anisomycin stabilizes the c-*fos* mRNA, extending the half-life from 30 min to between 4 and 6 hr.

4. A progressive shortening of c-*fos* mRNA occurs during degradation, probably because of a loss of 3′ poly(A) sequences.

Since agents as diverse as divalent calcium ions, mitogens like PDGF, and differentiation-specific agents like nerve growth factor (NGF) may induce *fos* gene expression, we began to search for a common pathway. Most of the agents that induce the c-*fos* gene seem also to activate protein kinase C.

Role of Protein Kinase C in the Activation of c-*fos* Expression

Protein kinase C is the receptor for the phorbol ester, TPA. Binding of TPA to protein kinase C activates the kinase activity of the receptor. In addition to TPA, the binding of growth factors to their receptors also activates protein kinase C. Since treatment of cells with appropriate growth factors or with TPA also results in increased expression of c-*fos,* one possible route to activating c-*fos* expression might involve the activation of protein kinase C. We studied the role of protein kinase C in induced expression of c-*fos* by stimulating protein kinase C with the calcium ionophore A23187 or DAG. We also tested the effect of DAG on c-*fos* expression in cells in which protein kinase C had been down-regulated by prolonged treatment with TPA.

RNA was first isolated from U-937 cells at intervals following addition of DAG to the culture (Fig. 8.3A). These cells responded by transiently synthesizing elevated levels of c-*fos* RNA, though expression of c-*fos* was alone insufficient to induce the differentiation of U-937 cells. When these cells were treated with A23187, they again expressed a transient burst of elevated c-*fos* RNA levels (Fig. 8.3B). In a similar fashion, rat 208F cells expressed a transient increase of c-*fos* RNA synthesis when treated with either TPA or DAG, but when pretreated for 60 hr with TPA at

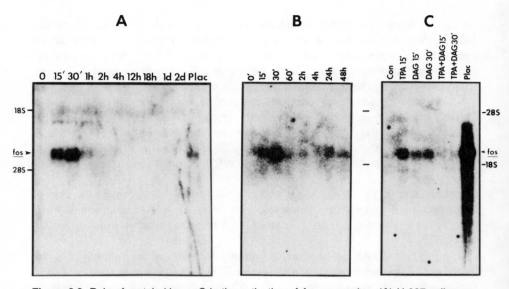

Figure 8.3. Role of protein kinase-C in the activation of *fos* expression. (**A**) U-937 cells were treated with diacylglycerol (OAG or DAG) and total RNA harvested following the time intervals indicated in the figure. RNA specific for the *fos* gene was detected by hybridization to a *fos* specific probe. (**B**) U-937 cells were treated with the calcium ionophore A-23187 (1 μM) and total RNA harvested at intervals as indicated. RNA specific for *fos* was detected as above. (**C**) RNA was isolated from untreated control (Con) rat 208F cells, from 208F cells treated with TPA or diacylglycerol (DAG, 25 μg/ml) for the times indicated, or from 208F cells treated with 100 nM TPA for 60 hr before treatment with DAG for the times indicated. *fos*-Specific RNA was detected by hybridization. Levels of *fos*-specific RNA are compared to the levels of *fos* detected in human placental RNA (Plac).

100 ng/ml to down-regulate protein kinase C, the cells became unresponsive to DAG treatment and failed to express c-*fos* (Fig. 8.3C). From this limited series of experiments it appears that the activation of protein kinase C may participate directly in activating the c-*fos* gene.

c-*fos* Expression during the Cell Cycle

The observation that *fos* expression is one of the earliest events to follow cell stimulation with either peptide growth factors or mitogens has led to the hypothesis that c-*fos* may be associated with specific cell cycle events. For example, *fos* might play a role in signal transduction during the normal cell cycle, or it might be associated only with such special circumstances as the transition from the quiescent (G_0) phase to the G_1 phase. We sought to determine if *fos* was expressed during the G_0/G_1 transition by studying the expression of *fos* following the synchronous release of HeLa cells from cell cycle arrest at the S or M phases of the cell cycle.

When we arrested HeLa cells by a double thymidine block, more than 95% of the cells were arrested in early S phase (Fig. 8.4A). When the cells were released from this metabolic block, c-*fos* RNA was synthesized in a typical rapid and transient burst (Fig. 8.4B) but was not elevated at any subsequent time. This increase of *fos*

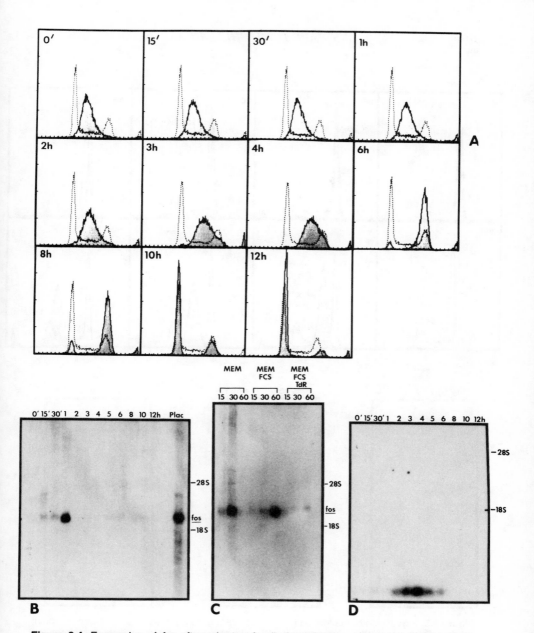

Figure 8.4. Expression of *fos* after release of cells from S-phase arrest induced by double thymidine block. HeLa cells were arrested during S phase by a double thymidine block as indicated in the text. At intervals following release from the second thymidine block, RNA was harvested at the times indicated (Panels B and C), and a sample of cells was subjected to flow-microfluorimetry to determine cell-cycle stage as indicated in the text. In Panel A, the sample cell population is shown by the shaded curve and a control population of cells during log-phase growth is shown by the dashed-line curve, with the left peak indicating the proportion of cells with 1N DNA content and the right peak indicating the proportion of cells with 2N DNA content. Specific RNA sequences were detected by hybridization to a *fos*-specific probe (Panel B) or a histone H2B specific probe (Panel C). Panel D, cells were released from the thymidine block into modified Eagle's medium lacking serum (MEM) or MEM with 10% fetal calf serum (MEM FCS) and 2mM thymidine (MEM FCS TdR). Human placental DNA sample is indicated (Plac)

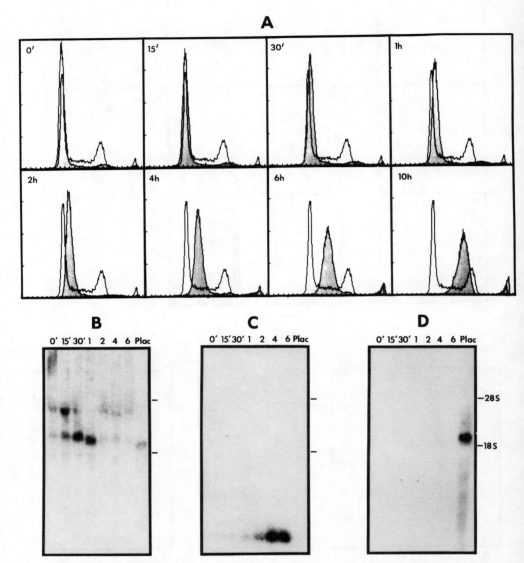

Figure 8.5. Expression of *fos* following release of cells from S-phase arrest induced by aphidi-colin or mitotic arrest induced by nitrous oxide. HeLa cells were arrested in S-phase by treatment with aphidicolin as indicated in the text (Panels A, B, C). Following release, RNA was harvested at intervals as indicated and specific sequences were detected with a *fos*-specific probe (B) or a histone H2B probe (C). Flow-microfluorimetry analysis is shown in Panel A. In Panel D, RNA was isolated at indicated intervals from HeLa cells after release from a mitotic arrest induced by cul-ture in high-pressure nitrous oxide, and RNA was detected by a *fos*-specific probe.

synthesis preceded the synthesis of histone H2B RNA (Fig. 8.4C). The expression of histone genes is known to correlate with the onset of DNA synthesis. The pattern of expression of c-*fos* after release from this S-phase block is not consistent with a direct role for c-*fos* in DNA synthesis. Furthermore, the expression of *fos* after release into medium lacking thymidine was not simply due to addition of fresh medium containing serum since release into medium lacking serum also results in *fos* expression (Fig. 8.4D). In fact, when the medium is simply replaced with fresh medium containing serum and thymidine, little increase in *fos* expression is observed (Fig. 8.4D).

Similarly, when cells blocked at the G_1/S boundary by treatment with aphidicolin

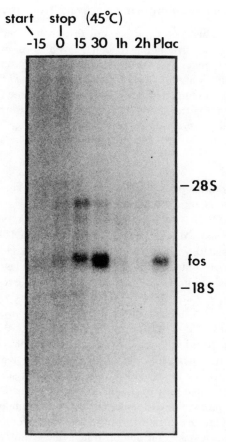

Figure 8.6. Expression of *fos* RNA during recovery of HeLa cells from heat shock. Cultures of HeLa cells were rapidly warmed to 45°C and maintained at this temperature for 15 min before rapid cooling to 37°C (stop, 0). RNA was harvested before heat shock (start, −15) and at the times indicated after stopping heat shock by cooling to 37°C. *fos*-specific sequences were detected in HeLa RNA samples and in a human placental RNA sample (Plac) by hybridization to a *fos*-specific probe.

are released synchronously, a transient burst of *fos* RNA synthesis is observed before the onset of histone H2B RNA synthesis (Figs. 8.5A and 8.5B). The *fos* gene, therefore, seems to be expressed as an early event following the release of a block of DNA synthesis. *fos* Induction appears to precede the induction of other genes involved in chromosome replication, for example, the histones.

To further examine the temporal expression of c-*fos* following release from cell cycle blockades, we arrested cells in mitotic metaphase by subjecting them to nitrous oxide under high pressure, a treatment that prevents spindle formation during mitosis. Figure 8.5D shows that no c-*fos* expression could be observed when the cells were released from the mitotic block. We conclude that *fos* expression is not required for completion of mitosis and progression through the early stages of G_1.

Expression of c-*fos* during Recovery from Heat Shock

Treatments that induce elevated expression of *fos,* such as serum stimulation, TPA treatment, and ultraviolet irradiation of cells, are also known to elevate the expression of heat shock genes. We therefore isolated RNA from HeLa cells at intervals following heat shock at 45°C for 15 min and determined the *fos* RNA levels by northern blot analysis. Figure 8.6 shows little or no *fos* gene induction during heat shock (level 2), but c-*fos* transcripts can be observed during recovery from heat shock. Once again, the expression is transient.

DISCUSSION

Expression of the proto-oncogene *fos* is one of the fastest known responses of cells to mitogens, growth factors and differentiation-inducing agents (Cochran et al. 1984, Greenberg and Ziff 1984, Kruijer et al. 1984, 1985, Muller et al. 1984a,b, 1985, Bravo et al. 1985, Mitchell et al. 1985, Treisman 1985). When quiescent fibroblasts are stimulated with PDGF, epidermal growth factor, serum, or TPA, c-*fos* transcripts are detected within minutes, and maximal levels accumulate within 30 to 60 min after induction. No c-*fos* transcripts are observed more than 120 min after induction (Kruijer et al. 1984).

In contrast, during TPA-induced differentiation of monomyelocytic cells to macrophages, the kinetics of c-*fos* transcription are different. While c-*fos* gene transcription is rapidly induced with maximal accumulation of c-*fos* transcripts within 30 to 60 min of TPA treatment, lower levels (about four- to fivefold lower than maximal levels) are detected for at least 109 hr after the initial stimulus (Mitchell et al. 1985). That no increase in c-*fos* expression accompanied the DMSO-induced differentiation of HL-60 promyelocytic leukemia cells to granulocytes suggested that c-*fos* expression might have a role in macrophage differentiation (Mitchell et al. 1985). More recently it has been demonstrated that expression of c-*fos* RNA in U-937 cells is insufficient to induce their differentiation to macrophages, and in some HL-60 variant cell lines, it is possible to induce differentiation to macrophages without increased expression of c-*fos* RNA, which suggests that *fos* may have a more general role (Mitchell et al. 1986).

Expression of c-*fos* may be modulated by activation of protein kinase C, a calcium and phospholipid-dependent enzyme that is activated by DAG. DAG is normally not found in high concentrations in membranes but is transiently produced from inositol phospholipids in response to several extracellular signals. TPA apparently activates protein kinase C by substituting for DAG (Nishizuka 1984). We reasoned that if c-*fos* expression is induced by TPA through activation of protein kinase C, then other agents that activate protein kinase C, such as DAG or calcium ionophores, should also stimulate it. Our evidence suggests that activation of protein kinase C provides at least one path to activation of c-*fos* expression since both DAG and A23187 increased the gene's expression. Furthermore, DAG-induced expression of c-*fos* is blocked by down-regulation of protein kinase C in rat 208F cells after prolonged incubation in the presence of 100 nM TPA. These results agree with those of Morgan and Curran (1986), who suggested that *fos* expression may be triggered directly through an activation of protein kinase C or through agents that open voltage-dependent calcium channels.

The observation that c-*fos* is expressed transiently following the serum-stimulated transition from the quiescent G_0 state to the G_1 phase of the cell cycle has led to speculation that *fos* expression might be correlated with specific cell cycle events. Our evidence demonstrating that *fos* expression also occurs following release from cells arrested in S phase suggests that *fos* expression is a more general response of cells to metabolic stimulation. This is further supported by the observation that *fos* expression occurs after release from a thymidine-induced S-phase arrest even in the absence of serum and that this expression is only slightly enhanced by medium change in the presence of thymidine. Our results extend the observations of Bravo et al. (1986), who reported that *fos* expression could be induced during any stage in the cell cycle except mitosis.

Eukaryotic and prokaryotic cells, when confronted with environmental stress, exhibit a reaction commonly called the "stress response." A diverse collection of treatments give rise to the stress response (for review see Ananthan et al. 1986, Ashburner and Bonner 1979). The *fos* gene product seems to be synthesized not in response to heat shock, but during recovery from heat shock. It is likely that *fos* expression is a general anabolic response of the cell to any external perturbation.

ACKNOWLEDGMENT

Richard L. Mitchell and Steven K. Hanks were supported by postdoctoral fellowships from the National Institutes of Health, F32GM 10161A and F32GM 09391, respectively. This research was supported by grants from the American Cancer Society and the National Cancer Institute to Inder M. Verma.

REFERENCES

Ananthan J, Goldberg AL, Voellmy R. 1986. Abnormal proteins serve as eukaryotic stress signals and trigger the activation of heat shock genes. Science 232:522–524.
Ashburner M, Bonner JJ. 1970. The induction of gene activity in Drosophila by heat shock. Cell 17:241–254.
Bishop JM. 1983. Cellular oncogenes and retroviruses. Annu Rev Biochem 52:301–354.

Bishop JM. 1985a. Trends in oncogenes. Trends in Genetics 1:245–249.

Bishop JM. 1985b. Viral oncogenes. Cell 42:23–38.

Bravo R, Burckhardt J, Curran T, Muller R. 1985. Stimulation and inhibition of growth by EGF in different A431 cell clones is accompanied by the rapid induction of c-*fos* and c-*myc* proto-oncogenes. EMBO J 4:1193–1197.

Bravo R, Burckhardt J, Curran T, Muller R. 1986. Expression of c-*fos* in NIH3T3 cells is very low but inducible throughout the cell cycle. EMBO J 5:695–700.

Chirgwin JM, Przybyla AE, MacDonald RJ, Rutter WJ. 1979. Isolation of biologically active ribonucleic acid from sources enriched in ribonuclease. Biochemistry 18:5294–5299.

Cochran BH, Zullo J, Verma IM, Stiles CD. 1984. Expression of the c-*fos* gene and of a *fos*-related gene is stimulated by platelet-derived growth factor. Science 226:1080–1082.

Cooper GM. 1982. Cellular transforming genes. Science 217:801–806.

Curran T, Verma IM. 1984. FBR murine osteosarcoma virus. I. Molecular analysis and characterization of a 75,000-Da *gag-fos* fusion product. Virology 135:218–228.

Curran T, Miller AD, Zokas L, Verma IM. 1984. Viral and cellular *fos* proteins: A comparative analysis. Cell 36:259–268.

Curran T, Peters G, Van Beveren C, Teich NM, Verma IM. 1982. The FBJ murine osteosarcoma virus: Identification and molecular cloning of biologically active proviral DNA. J Virol 44:674–682.

Curran T, Teich NM. 1982. Product of the FBJ murine osteosarcoma virus oncogene: Characterization of a 55,000 dalton phosphoprotein. J Virol 42:114–122.

Doolittle RF, Hunkapillar MW, Hood LE, et al. 1983. Simian sarcoma virus *onc* gene (or genes) encoding a platelet derived growth factor. Science 221:275–277.

Finkel MP, Biskis BO, Jinkins PB. 1966. Virus induction of osteosarcomas in mice. Science 151:698–701.

Finkel MP, Reilly CA, Biskis BO, Greco JL. 1972. Bone tumor viruses. *In* Colson Papers, Proceedings of the 24th Symposium of the Colson Research Society, pp 353–366.

Gonda TJ, Metcalf D. 1984. Expression of *myb, myc* and *fos* proto-oncogenes during the differentiation of a murine myeloid leukaemia. Nature 310:249–251.

Gray JW, Coffino P. 1979. Cell cycle analysis by flow cytometry. Methods Enzymol 58:233–262.

Greenberg ME, Ziff EB. 1984. Stimulation of 3T3 cells induces transcription of the c-*fos* proto-oncogene. Nature 311:433–438.

Greenberg ME, Hermanowski AL, Ziff EB. 1985. Effect of protein synthesis inhibitors on growth factor activation of c-*fos*, c-*myc* and actin gene transcription. Mol Cell Biol 6:1050–1057.

Hunter T. 1984. The proteins of oncogenes. Sci Am 251:70–79.

Kruijer W, Cooper JA, Hunter T, Verma IM. 1984. Platelet-derived growth factor induces rapid but transient expression of the c-*fos* gene and protein. Nature 312:711–716.

Kruijer W, Schubert D, Verma IM. 1985. Induction of the proto-oncogene *fos* by nerve growth factor. Proc Natl Acad Sci USA 82:7330–7334.

Lehrach H, Diamond D, Wozney JM, Boedtker H. 1977. RNA molecular weight determinations by gel electrophoresis under denaturing conditions, a critical re-examination. Biochemistry 16:4743–4751.

MacConnell WP, Verma IM. 1983. Expression of FBJ-MSV oncogene (*fos*) product in bacteria. Virology 131:367–374.

Meijlink F, Curran T, Miller AD, Verma IM. 1985. Removal of a 67 base pair sequence in the non-coding region of proto-oncogene *fos* converts it to a transforming gene. Proc Natl Acad Sci USA 82:4987–4991.

Meinkoth J, Wahl G. 1984. Hybridization of nucleic acids immobilized on solid supports. Anal Biochem 138:267–284.

Miller AD, Curran T, Verma IM. 1984. c-*fos* Protein can induce cellular transformation: A novel mechanism of activation of a cellular oncogene. Cell 36:51–60.

Mitchell RL, Henning-Chubb C, Huberman E, Verma IM. 1986. c-*fos* Expression is neither sufficient nor obligatory for differentiation of monomyelocytes to macrophages. Cell 45:497–504.

Mitchell RL, Zokas L, Schreiber RD, Verma IM. 1985. Rapid induction of the expression of proto-oncogene *fos* during human monocytic differentiation. Cell 40:209–217.

Morgan JI, Curran T. 1986. Role of ion flux in the control of c-*fos* expression. Nature 322:552–555.

Muller R, Bravo R, Burckhardt J, Curran T. 1984a. Induction of c-*fos* gene and protein by growth factors precedes activation of c-*myc*. Nature 312:716–720.

Muller R, Curran T, Muller D, Guilbert L. 1985. Induction of c-*fos* during myelomonocytic differentiation and macrophage proliferation. Nature 314:546–548.

Muller R, Muller D, Guilbert L. 1984b. Differential expression of c-*fos* during myelomono-cytic differentiation and macrophage proliferation. EMBO J 3:1887–1890.

Muller R, Slamon DJ, Tremblay JM, Cline MJ, Verma IM. 1982. Differential expression of cellular oncogenes during pre- and postnatal development of the mouse. Nature 299:640–644.

Muller R, Verma IM. 1984. Expression of cellular oncogenes. Curr Top Microbiol Immunol 112:73–115.

Nishizuka Y. 1984. The role of protein kinase C in cell surface signal transduction and tu-mour promotion. Nature 308:693–698.

Rao PN. 1968. Mitotic synchrony in mammalian cells treated with nitrous oxide at high pres-sure. Science 160:774–776.

Rigby PWJ, Diechmann M, Rhodes C, Berg P. 1977. Labeling deoxyribonucleic acid to high specific activity in vitro by nick translation with DNA polymerase I. J Mol Biol 113:237–251.

Ross R, Raines EW, Bowen-Pope DF. 1986. The biology of platelet-derived growth factor. Cell 46:155–169.

Sherr CJ, Rettenmier CW, Sacca R, Roussel MF, Look AT, Stanley ER. 1985. The c-*fms* proto-oncogene product is related to the receptor for the mononuclear phagocyte growth factor, CSF-1. Cell 41:665–676.

Sundstrom C, Nilsson K. 1976. Establishment and characterization of a human histiocytic lymphoma cell line (U-937). Int J Cancer 17:565–577.

Thomas PS. 1980. Hybridization of denatured RNA and small DNA fragments transferred to nitrocellulose. Proc Natl Acad Sci USA 77:5201–5205.

Treisman R. 1985. Transient accumulation of c-*fos* RNA following serum stimulation re-quires a conserved 5′ element and c-*fos* 3′ sequences. Cell 42:889–902.

Van Beveren C, Enami S, Curran T, Verma IM. 1984. FBR murine osteosarcoma virus. II. Nucleotide sequence of the provirus reveals that the genome contains sequences acquired from two cellular genes. Virology 135:229.

Van Beveren C, van Straaten F, Curran T, Muller R, Verma IM. 1983. Analysis of FBJ-MuSV provirus and c-*fos* (mouse) gene reveals that viral and cellular *fos* gene products have dif-ferent carboxy termini. Cell 32:1241–1255.

van Straaten F, Muller R, Curran T, Verma IM. 1983. Complete nucleotide sequence of a human c-*onc* gene: Deduced amino acid sequence of the human c-*fos* protein. Proc Natl Acad Sci USA 80:3183.

Verma IM, Curran T, Muller R, et al. 1984. The *fos* gene: Organization and expression. *In* Cancer Cells 2/Oncogenes and Viral Genes. Cold Spring Harbor Press, New York, pp. 309–321.

Waterfield MD, Scrace GT, Whittle N, et al. 1983. Platelet-derived growth factor is struc-turally related to the putative transforming protein p28^{sis} of simian sarcoma virus. Nature 304:35.

Weinberg RA. 1983. A molecular basis of cancer. Sci Am 249:126–142.

Symposium on Fundamental Cancer Research, Vol. 39.
© 1987 by The University of Texas System Cancer Center.

9. Genetic Sequences That Predispose to Retinoblastoma and Osteosarcoma

Thaddeus P. Dryja, Stephen Friend,* and Robert A. Weinberg*

*Department of Ophthalmology, Massachusetts Eye and Ear Infirmary
and Harvard Medical School, Boston, Massachusetts 02115
and * Whitehead Institute for Biomedical Research and Department of Biology,
Massachusetts Institute of Technology, Cambridge, Massachusetts 02142*

The genetic predisposing factor for childhood retinoblastoma resides on the q14 band of human chromosome 13. However, a postulated second genetic event must take place for the disease to occur, which further research indicates involves inactivation of the remaining functional allele within 13q14.

Our isolation of the gene within 13q14, called Rb, required creating a lambda-phage library that contained inserted fragments from human chromosome 13. One of the inserts, H3-8, detected a corresponding 1.8-kb HindIII fragment that was deleted in 2 of 37 retinoblastoma tumor DNAs. This suggested that the probed segment was linked to the Rb gene. A nearby probe, p7H30.7R, detected not only the human sequence but also a mouse homologue in a somatic cell hybrid carrying human chromosome 13.

We used the p7H30.7R probe for RNA analysis to detect any transcripts in a retinal cell line. The analysis showed a 4.7-kb transcript in the tumor cell line but not in several retinoblastomas. We also failed to detect a transcript in four retinoblastoma and two osteosarcoma samples using a corresponding cDNA fragment termed p4.7R. We used this probe to analyze the DNA from a large group of retinoblastomas and osteosarcomas and found gross changes in genomic structure in approximately 30% of the tumor DNAs. The boundaries of homozygously deleted fragments were mapped. In the analysis of an osteosarcoma and a retinoblastoma we discovered that the endpoints of the deletions were within the confines of the genetic unit defined by the probe. This indicated that the target of inactivation was the segment under study and not a neighboring DNA sequence.

Until 10 years ago, the mechanisms of human carcinogenesis were studied at the level of cell and organism with only distant reference to the genetic elements underlying the observed processes. In 1976, the first genetic element that can affect carcinogenesis was described. In that year, the research group of Varmus and Bishop uncovered the *src* proto-oncogene, an element of the normal vertebrate genome that acquires oncogenic powers upon association with an avian retrovirus (Stehelin et al. 1976). This work established the paradigm that normal cellular genes may undergo mutations that allow them to induce the malignant conversion of cells in which they arise.

To be sure, these initial experiments only addressed proto-oncogenes that are activated by retrovirus genomes. Within six years, it became apparent, however, that somatic mutational processes that are independent of viruses may also succeed in activating these genes to an oncogenic state. The number of isolated cellular proto-oncogenes and derived oncogenes now approaches 30, a third of which have been found in altered form in human tumor DNAs (Bishop 1983, Varmus 1984).

These oncogenes constitute a diverse array, in that their gene products are localized to a variety of subcellular sites and act by a number of distinct mechanisms (Land et al. 1983). But they share one trait: they all act in a genetically dominant manner in the cell. Thus, whether these oncogenes arise endogenously by alteration of a cell's genome or are introduced into a cell by a viral vector or gene transfer, they act to change the cell's phenotype even in the presence of related wild-type alleles.

A second, less documented attribute may be shared by these oncogenes. Their involvement in human tumorigenesis seems to follow events of somatic mutation. As such, they reflect genetic damage that occurs during an individual's lifetime but they do not reflect genetic elements that are transmitted from one generation to the next.

We have been studying a human tumor of childhood that often appears as a consequence of an underlying, familial predisposition. That a predisposition to childhood retinoblastoma can be an inherited trait has been postulated for much of this century. Indeed, hereditary transmission of this trait was already observed almost a century ago (deGouvea 1910).

Within the past decade, this genetic predisposing factor was localized to a single discrete band of human chromosome 13. The localization depended in large part on karyotypic studies of the tumors and normal tissues of afflicted individuals. In some cases, a variety of inherited balanced translocations was observed. Although they reached to various extents over the long arm of chromosome 13, these deletions invariably involved the q14 band (Gilbert 1986).

At the same time, it became apparent that such karyotypic abnormalities could be inherited from a parent, arise during gametogenesis, or develop somatically. The end result was the same—loss of one copy of a gene or genes in this chromosomal band. Yet this model did not entirely explain the etiology of the disease. As Knudson realized, although all the retinal cells of a congenitally affected child may bear an inactivated 13q14 allele, only a small number of these cells undergo malignant conversion. Accordingly, he postulated that a second genetic event, acting in concert with the initial one, intervened to spawn tumorigenic progeny (Knudson 1971).

Other work has subsequently made it apparent that this second event involves inactivation of the remaining, hitherto functional allele at 13q14. This was shown by studying the behavior of genetically linked markers, including the esterase D gene and certain restriction fragment-length polymorphisms (RFLP). These markers, which were often found in a heterozygous state in the unaffected tissues of a patient, were seen frequently in a homozygous state in the tumor. This indicated that the surviving normal allele is often replaced by its inactive counterpart during tumorigenesis (Godbout et al. 1983, Cavenee et al. 1983, Dryja et al. 1984).

Taken together, these results leave several conclusions for those studying the genetic basis of this disease. First, the 13q14 gene, often termed Rb, seems to influence tumorigenesis only upon inactivation of both homologous normal alleles. Consequently, the mutant alleles are unable to elicit phenotypic change in the presence of corresponding normal, wild-type alleles. Second, sometimes the Rb gene is inactivated by a deletion of its DNA sequence, causing tumors occasionally to suffer homozygous deletion during tumorigenesis. Homozygous deletions, in turn, should provide a critical molecular landmark in a study seeking to define the limits of this gene and to isolate its normal version by molecule cloning.

Initial steps toward the isolation of the Rb gene depended upon the creation of a lambdaphage library that contained inserted fragments originating from human chromosome 13. This was accomplished by use of a fluorescence-activated cell sorter that allowed the enrichment of chromosome 13 from a mixture of metaphase chromosomes. These experiments led to the isolation of a number of lambdaphage carrying chromosome 13 inserts (Lalande et al. 1984). These inserts were then mapped to various regions of chromosome 13, two DNA fragments being mapped to 13q14. One of these, termed H3-8, was especially interesting. When used in the analysis of 37 retinoblastoma tumor DNAs, it detected a corresponding 1.8-kb *Hin*dIII fragment in all but two of these. These two tumor DNAs totally lacked the 1.8-kb fragment because it had undergone homozygous deletion. The nontumor DNA of these patients did not have these deletions, which showed that this homozygous deletion occurred as a consequence of somatic mutation (Dryja et al. 1986).

These observations suggested that the genomic DNA segment recognized by the probe was closely linked to the Rb gene. Large chromosome 13 deletions (i.e., those detectable cytogenetically) are never observed in a homozygous state in retinoblastoma cells, indicating that nullizygosity of only a small portion of chromosome 13 is tolerated by the tumor cells. This in turn suggested that any sequence—like the one detected by the H3-8 probe—that undergoes homozygous deletion is tightly linked to the Rb locus.

Another finding prompted us to characterize further the DNA sequence linked to the H3-8 probe. When a nearby probe p7H30.7R was used to analyze DNA of the somatic cell hybrid carrying human chromosome 13, it detected the expected human sequence as well as a mouse homologue. Such a result showed a substantial evolutionary conservation of this sequence, a finding that often indicates the presence of a protein-encoding sequence.

Accordingly, we used the p7H30.7R probe in northern (i.e., RNA) blot analyses in an attempt to detect any transcripts that may derive from this region. We surveyed the RNA of several retinoblastoma tumor cell lines. As control, we used a human retinal cell line that had been immortalized after transfection of adenovirus DNA. This cell line presumably suffered no genetic changes at the Rb locus. The northern blots showed a 4.7-kb transcript that was present in the tumor cell line and absent from several retinoblastoma samples. This was compatible with an association between this transcript and the Rb gene that we presumed to be inactive in these tumor cells (Friend et al. 1986).

A cDNA library was constructed using the RNA of the retinal cell line. Screening of this library with the probe yielded a clone, termed p4.7R, which appears to carry virtually all the sequence information that is present in the 4.7-kb mRNA. When we used fragments derived from this clone as probes in northern blot analysis, we once again failed to detect a transcript in four retinoblastomas as well as in two osteosarcoma samples. The RNAs of the latter were analyzed because these bone tumors are often seen in individuals who carry alterations of the Rb locus (Draper et al. 1986).

Next we used this probe to study by Southern blot analysis the DNAs of a large group of retinoblastomas and osteosarcomas. The p4.7R probe was seen to survey a genomic region of more than 70 kb, a region that has a complex structure with at least six exons.

These DNA analyses revealed gross changes in genomic structure in approximately 30% of the tumor DNAs, changes manifested as underrepresented fragments, fragments of altered length, and totally absent fragments. Since homozygously deleted fragments were the most informative, we mapped the boundaries of these deletions. At least four tumors were found to have undergone deletions that began within the surveyed region and extended to the left on the genome map that we constructed independently. Although encouraging, this result was hardly definitive; it might indicate that the Rb gene lay somewhere to the left, being inactivated by deletions that incidentally included neighboring genes such as the one we were studying.

The critical results came after analysis of the DNAs of an osteosarcoma and a retinoblastoma. In these cases, the observed deletions had endpoints that were totally within the confines of the genetic unit defined by the probe. This showed that the critical target of inactivation was the segment under study and not a neighboring DNA sequence.

Although these data strongly support the identity of this segment with the Rb locus, they leave many questions unanswered. The transcript of this gene is apparently absent from some tumors that have no gross alterations in the sequences of this region. Of even greater importance are the issues concerning the gene's mechanisms of action. How does it function in normal ontogeny, and how does its absence predispose specifically to retinoblastomas and osteosarcomas? These issues have not been addressed in even a preliminary fashion to date, and their resolution will require great effort in the years ahead.

REFERENCES

Bishop JM. 1983. Cellular oncogenes and retroviruses. Annu Rev Biochem 52:301–354.
Cavenee WK, Dryja TP, Phillips RA, et al. 1983. Expression of recessive alleles by chromosomal mechanisms in retinoblastoma. Nature 305:779–784.
deGouvea H. 1910. L'hérédité des gliomes de la rétine. Annales d'Oculistique 143:32–34.
Draper GJ, Sanders BM, Kingston JE. 1986. Second primary neoplasms in patients with retinoblastoma. Br J Cancer 53:661–663.
Dryja TP, Cavenee W, White R, et al. 1984. Homozygosity of chromosome 13 in retinoblastoma. N Engl J Med 310:550–553.
Dryja TP, Rapaport JM, Joyce JM, Petersen RA. 1986. Molecular detection of deletions involving band q14 of chromosome 13 in retinoblastomas. Proc Natl Acad Sci USA 83:7391–7394.

Friend SH, Bernards R, Rogelj S, et al. 1986. A human DNA segment with properties of the gene that predisposes to retinoblastoma and osteosarcoma. Nature 323:643–646.

Gilbert F. 1986. Retinoblastoma and cancer genetics. N Engl J Med 314:1248–1250.

Godbout R, Dryja TP, Squire J, Gallie BL, Phillips RA. 1983. Somatic inactivation of genes on chromosome 13 is a common event in retinoblastoma. Nature 304:451–453.

Knudson AG Jr. 1971. Mutation and cancer: Statistical study of retinoblastoma. Proc Natl Acad Sci USA 68:280–283.

Lalande M, Dryja TP, Schreck RR, Shipley J, Flint A, Latt SA. 1984. Isolation of human chromosome 13-specific DNA sequences cloned from flow sorted chromosomes and potentially linked to the retinoblastoma locus. Cancer Genet Cytogenet 13:283–295.

Land H, Parada LF, Weinberg RA. 1983. Cellular oncogenes and multistep carcinogenesis. Science 222:771–778.

Stehelin D, Varmus HE, Bishop JM, Vogt PK. 1976. DNA related to transforming gene(s) of avian sarcoma viruses is present in normal avian DNA. Nature 260:170–173.

Varmus HE. 1984. The molecular genetics of cellular oncogenes. Annu Rev Genet 18:553–612.

ONCOGENE FUNCTION: THE *RAS* MODEL

Symposium on Fundamental Cancer Research, Vol. 39.
© 1987 by The University of Texas System Cancer Center.

10. Guanine Nucleotide-Binding Proteins Involved in Transmembrane Signaling

Eva J. Neer

Cardiovascular Division, Department of Medicine,
Brigham and Women's Hospital and Harvard Medical School,
Boston, Massachusetts 02115

Transmission of signals from a hormone-receptor complex to a number of intra-cellular effectors is mediated by a family of guanine nucleotide-binding proteins (G proteins). Each G protein consists of an α, β, and γ subunit and is most clearly distinguished from other G proteins by the biological and biochemical attributes of its GTP-binding α subunit. The α proteins can be divided into general classes by their susceptibility to modification by the bacterial toxins, cholera toxin, and pertussis toxin.

In brain, there are three substrates for ADP-ribosylation by pertussis toxin with molecular weights of 41,000 (α_{41}), 40,000 (α_{40}) and 39,000 (α_{39}). The α_{39} is the most abundant. We purified the α_{41} and α_{39} proteins from bovine brain and have used immunologic and biochemical tools to compare their structure and function. We have also isolated and characterized a cDNA clone from a bovine pituitary library that encodes α_{41}. The deduced amino acid sequence of the α_{41} clone demonstrates marked homology to several other GTP-binding proteins. Southern blot analysis of the cloned α_{41} cDNA suggests the presence of two genes encoding this G protein. In addition, we identified a cDNA clone for a novel, putative G protein, α_{h}, which demonstrates marked sequence homology with other G proteins but which repre-sents a clearly distinct gene product. Taken together, these data suggest a new level of complexity in the organization of the G protein supergene family, with multiple G proteins of similar overall structural and mechanistic properties likely to be identi-fied as products of distinct genes.

The transmembrane signaling system for many hormones and neurotransmitters consists of three parts, the input mechanism (hormone receptor), the output mecha-nism (adenylate cyclase, phospholipases, ion channels) and the coupling system that links them. For many hormones and neurotransmitters, the coupling proteins are a set of heterotrimeric guanine nucleotide-binding proteins (G proteins) made up of α, β, and γ subunits. These coupling proteins affect the function of both the output and the input systems. When GTP or a nonhydrolyzable GTP analogue such as guanosine 5'-(3-O-thio) triphosphate (GTPγS) or guanosine 5'-(β,γ-imino)triphos-phate (Gpp(NH)p) is bound to the G protein, the receptor's affinity for the hormone is diminished (Lefkowitz et al. 1982). A great deal of evidence shows that this modulation is mediated by the formation of a ternary complex between the hormone receptor and a guanine nucleotide-binding protein (deLean et al. 1980). Thus, sensitivity to guanine nucleotide is a characteristic feature of hormone receptors that send signals across the plasma membrane by the G proteins.

The hormone receptors linked to G proteins fall into three categories: those that activate adenylate cyclase, those that inhibit adenylate cyclase, and those that exert their actions by mechanisms that do not involve changes in cyclic nucleotide levels. Many hormones can act in all three ways, however. Catecholamines, for example, acting through β-adrenergic receptors, stimulate adenylate cyclase (Lefkowitz et al. 1982), acting through α_2 receptors, inhibit adenylate cyclase (Steer and Wood 1979, Hoffman et al. 1982), and acting through α_1 receptors, change cellular metabolism by affecting phosphoinositol turnover (Burch et al. 1986). Such observations raise several fundamental questions. Are there many G proteins, with each receptor linked to a different one, or are there a few G proteins that interact with classes of receptors or classes of effectors? These questions have been only partly answered, and they are the subject of intense investigation by many research groups.

FUNCTIONS OF G PROTEINS

The G proteins, which mediate hormone responses, may be divided into two broad classes according to their interaction with the bacterial toxins from *Vibrio cholera* and *Bordetella pertussis*. These bacterial toxins are enzymes that transfer ADP-ribose from NAD to the α subunit of the G proteins. This activity has been of enormous practical importance since it allowed the first radioactive labeling of the α proteins so they could be identified in membranes and studied long before they were actually purified (Gill and Meren 1978). The G proteins involved in hormonal stimulation of adenylate cyclase are substrates for cholera toxin (Gill and Meren 1978, Cassel and Pfeuffer 1978), whereas those involved in hormonal inhibition of adenylate cyclase and in regulation of other enzymes (see below) are substrates for pertussis toxin (Katada and Ui 1982, Ui et al. 1984). In addition, transducin, a related protein from retinal rod outer segments, is a substrate for modification by both toxins (Van Dop et al. 1984a,b). All these proteins are heterotrimers composed of α, β, and γ subunits and have been purified from several sources. The α subunits have many properties in common which are summarized in Table 10.1.

The α subunits bind guanine nucleotides, both GTP and its nonhydrolyzable analogues such as Gpp(NH)p or GTPγS (Smigel et al. 1984). The naturally occurring nucleotide GTP activates the α subunit only transiently because the α subunit has a GTPase activity that cleaves GTP to the inactive guanine nucleotide, GDP (Cassel and Selinger 1976, Pederson and Ross 1982, Neer et al. 1984, Sunyer et al. 1984). Nonhydrolyzable GTP analogues (GTPγS, Gpp(NH)p), in contrast, activate the α subunit for a long time (Londos et al. 1974). Resolved α subunits have been shown to interact directly with hormone receptors to modulate their affinity for ligands (Pederson and Ross 1982). Conversely, pure hormone receptors can enhance the GTPase activity of pure α proteins (Pederson and Ross 1982, Brandt et al. 1983).

Table 10.1. *Properties of α Subunits*

Bind guanine nucleotides
Hydrolyze GTP
Reversibly associate with $\beta \cdot \gamma$
Modified by bacterial toxins
Interact with receptors
Interact with effectors (enzymes, channels)
Many different proteins

In solution, the $\alpha \cdot \beta \cdot \gamma$ heterotrimer is dissociated by nonhydrolyzable guanine nucleotides (Northup et al. 1983a,b, Codina et al. 1984, Katada et al. 1984, Huff et al. 1985, Neer et al. 1987) into α and $\beta \cdot \gamma$, the $\beta \cdot \gamma$ subunits do not dissociate into monomers except under denaturing conditions. GTP does not cause dissociation of at least one kind of $\alpha \cdot \beta \cdot \gamma$ heterotrimer (Huff et al. 1985). It is not yet clear whether this failure to dissociate the heterotrimer is the result of GTP hydrolysis to GDP (a nondissociating ligand) by the GTPase activity inherent in the α protein or the result of GTP's being less effective than GTPγS or Gpp(NH)p in dissociating the subunits. Clearly, we must learn which alternative is true to understand the role of subunit dissociation in membranes.

ACTIVATION OF ADENYLATE CYCLASE

In some cases, the α proteins have been shown to interact directly with the effector enzymes. One of the best studied examples is the interaction of the stimulatory α component, α_s, with the catalytic unit of adenylate cyclase. The currently accepted model for activating adenylate cyclase, at least in solution, is shown in Figure 10.1 (Smigel et al. 1984). The nonhydrolyzable guanine nucleotides dissociate α from the $\beta \cdot \gamma$ subunit. The guanine nucleotide liganded α protein then interacts directly with the catalytic unit of adenylate cyclase to activate it. The model is supported by the observation that GTPγS-liganded α_s, separated from $\beta \cdot \gamma$, is sufficient to activate the catalytic unit (Northup et al. 1983b). Furthermore, upon activation, the size of the catalytic unit increases by 50 kDa, the approximate molecular mass of α_s which is consistent with direct association of α_s with the enzyme (Bender et al. 1984). Reconstitution of the stimulatory G protein, G_s, with the catalytic unit of adenylate cyclase is quite straightforward and does not require phospholipid vesicles.

The model shown in Figure 10.1 predicts the effect of $\beta \cdot \gamma$ on activation because increasing the concentration of $\beta \cdot \gamma$ will shift the equilibrium shown to the left; that is, to the deactivated form of G_s. In fact, in an in vitro reconstituted system, one can demonstrate the predicted effect of $\beta \cdot \gamma$. In our hands (Neer et al. 1987) and in the work reported by Northup et al. (1983a) $\beta \cdot \gamma$ has no direct inhibitory effect on the adenylate cyclase catalytic unit, provided that the catalytic unit preparation is free of contaminating α_s.

The availability of the purified components allows one to ask whether or not a pure hormone receptor, guanine nucleotide-binding protein, and a catalytic unit, are sufficient to reconstitute hormonally responsive adenylate cyclase; the answer is

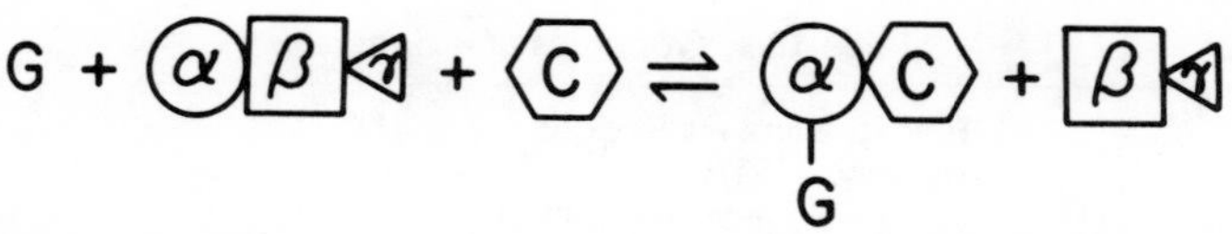

$$G + \textcircled{α}\boxed{\beta}\boxed{\triangleleft} + \langle C \rangle \rightleftharpoons \textcircled{α}\langle C \rangle + \boxed{\beta}\boxed{\triangleleft}$$
$$\underset{G}{\mid}$$

Figure 10.1. Model for activation of adenylate cyclase. G, a guanine nucleotide triphosphate; α, β, γ, the subunits of the stimulatory G protein; C, the catalytic unit of adenylate cyclase.

yes. The catalytic unit of adenylate cyclase, partially purified from bovine brain, was reconstituted in phospholipid vesicles with G_s purified from human erythrocytes and a β-adrenergic receptor purified from guinea pig lung (Cerione et al. 1984), showing that these three components are indeed sufficient for a hormonal response. A phospholipid vesicle is necessary for the reconstitution. The exact orientation of the components in the vesicle is not yet known. Both catalytic units and hormone receptors are hydrophobic, intrinsic membrane proteins that probably span the lipid bilayer. The $\beta\cdot\gamma$ proteins are quite hydrophobic (Huff et al. 1985, Sternweis 1986) and may act as the membrane anchor for the α proteins (Sternweis 1986). The success of the reconstitution experiment suggests that the interfaces among the components are extraordinarily conserved because the receptor, the guanine nucleotide-binding proteins, and the catalytic unit all came from different tissues and species. The interchangeability of the subunits also argues for the generality of the mechanism of activation.

Although the mechanism of activation has been well demonstrated in solution, it is not yet certain that the $\alpha_s\cdot\beta\cdot\gamma$ heterotrimer actually dissociates in the membrane nor that α_s dissociates from C. If dissociation were involved in hormonal activation of adenylate cyclase, then complex kinetics of activation would be expected. However, Tolkovsky et al. (1982) observed that hormonal activation is a first-order process and that the first-order rate constant depends on the receptor concentration. They suggested, therefore, that α_s and the catalytic unit are permanently coupled in the membrane. This issue is still not definitively resolved.

OTHER FUNCTIONS OF THE α AND $\beta\cdot\gamma$ SUBUNITS

There is more agreement about the mechanism of activation of adenylate cyclase than about the mechanism of hormonal inhibition of adenylate cyclase or of hormonal control of noncyclic AMP-mediated functions. Hormonal inhibition of adenylate cyclase is mediated by a guanine nucleotide-binding protein different from the protein that mediates the stimulatory response. Two possible models for the mechanism of hormonal inhibition of adenylate cyclase are shown in Figure 10.2. The first model is directly analogous to the model for hormonal stimulation. The $\alpha_i\cdot\beta\cdot\gamma$ heterotrimer is dissociated by guanine nucleotides (as shown by hydrodynamic studies), and the guanine nucleotide-liganded α component interacts directly with the catalytic unit, except instead of stimulation, this association causes inhibition. Another mechanism (proposed by Smigel et al. 1984) is based on the consequence of the fact that both stimulatory and inhibitory guanine nucleotide-

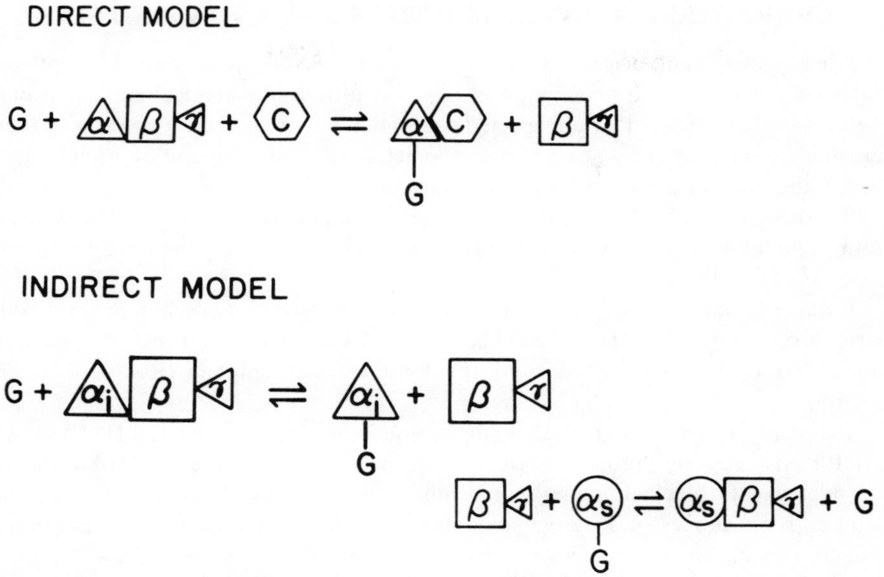

DIRECT MODEL

INDIRECT MODEL

Figure 10.2. Models for inhibition of adenylate cyclase. G, a guanine nucleotide triphosphate; α_s, the α component of the stimulatory G protein; α_i the α component of the inhibitory G protein; C, the catalytic unit of adenylate cyclase.

binding proteins share a common $\beta \cdot \gamma$ subunit. In this mechanism, inhibition is not direct but occurs by turning off the activation process. Dissociation of α_i from $\beta \cdot \gamma$ increases the concentration of $\beta \cdot \gamma$, which shifts the equilibrium of α_s and $\beta \cdot \gamma$ toward the associated or inactive form, and therefore reverses activation of the catalytic unit. There is evidence for both mechanisms. Increasing the concentration of $\beta \cdot \gamma$ has been shown to deactivate G_s (Northup et al. 1983, Neer et al. 1987). Furthermore, for the indirect mechanism to work α_i must be in excess over α_s so that it can act as a reservoir for a considerable amount of $\beta \gamma$. Otherwise, dissociation of α_i from $\beta \cdot \gamma$ would not cause a substantial increase in the $\beta \cdot \gamma$ concentration. The relative amounts of the subunits have not been measured in many tissues, but in brain α_i seems to be in excess over α_s (Huff and Neer 1986). Some observations cannot, however, be explained by the indirect model, which would predict that in the absence of G_s, there should be no hormonal inhibition. Genetically deficient cells that are totally lacking in α_s (Harris et al. 1985) provide a test system. In these cells, one would expect no hormonal inhibition of adenylate cyclase, yet hormonal inhibition has been demonstrated (Hildebrandt and Birnbaumer 1983). It is possible, therefore, that direct inhibition of the catalytic unit by α_i occurs in these cells. The exact balance of these mechanisms in any particular intact cell has not yet been defined.

According to the preceding discussions the active component is the α subunit while the $\beta \cdot \gamma$ unit has an inhibitory role. Recently, however, Logothetis et al. (1987) showed that the purified $\beta \cdot \gamma$ subunit can activate the K^+ channel in chick atrial cells. Thus, dissociation of the $\alpha \cdot \beta \cdot \gamma$ heterotrimer may result in two active species.

CHARACTERIZATION OF MULTIPLE α, β, AND γ PROTEINS

All these considerations were fairly straightforward as long as we thought there was fundamentally one kind of α_s, α_i, and $\beta \cdot \gamma$. Yet further biochemical and molecular genetic studies revealed an unexpected multiplicity of α, β, and γ proteins. There are at least two kinds of γ protein, one associated with the β subunit of retinal transducin and another associated with the β subunit of G proteins (Hildebrandt et al. 1985). Fong et al. (1986) recently cloned cDNA encoding the β subunit from bovine retina and found at least two forms of β-related mRNAs in many mammalian tissues and clonal cell lines.

It has been known for many years that most cells contain two cholera toxin substrates, one of 52–55 kDa and another of 42–45 kDa. The two forms of α_s may be derived from a single mRNA transcript by alternative splicing (Robishaw et al. 1986b).

Originally, α_i was thought to be a single protein because a single 41-kDa band was ADP-ribosylated by pertussis toxin in most cell types, and the ADP-ribosylation correlated with blockade of hormonal inhibition of adenylate cyclase. Functional studies soon suggested heterogeneity, however, because a number of hormonal effects, which were not mediated by changes in cyclic nucleotide levels, were blocked by pertussis toxin. The blockade correlated with ADP-ribosylation of a 41-kDa membrane protein (Bokoch and Gilman 1984). The question then became whether one protein mediates both inhibition of adenylate cyclase and modulation of other enzymes or whether there are multiple pertussis toxin substrates. The answer began to emerge with the discovery that in some tissues, at least, there are multiple substrates for ADP-ribosylation. In brain, for example, we found three distinct substrates for ADP-ribosylation with molecular masses of 41 kDa, 40 kDa, and 39 kDa (Neer et al. 1984). We purified two of them, the 41-kDa and 39-kDa proteins and called them α_{41} and α_{39}. These proteins were independently purified by Sternweis and Robishaw (1984) who called them α_i and α_o respectively. The 40-kDa protein is the least abundant and has not yet been completely purified. What is the relation of these three proteins? We raised a polyclonal antibody to the 39-kDa protein and found that the antibody recognizes α_{39} much better than it recognizes α_{41}, although there is a small amount of cross-reactivity (Huff and Neer 1986). These results show that the proteins are related but α_{39} cannot be a proteolytic fragment of α_{41}. As will be discussed below, there is direct evidence from the sequence of the cloned cDNAs corresponding to these proteins that they are, in fact, different gene products. The availability of antibodies allowed us to determine how much α_{39} protein there is in bovine brain. We were surprised to find that the protein makes up about 0.5% of total brain membrane protein, although this is consistent with our yields on purification. We also made antibodies to the brain $\beta \cdot \gamma$ protein and were able to show that, although the sum of all the α proteins is a substantial fraction of membrane protein, there is nevertheless enough $\beta \cdot \gamma$ to match the amount of α. Although the α_{39} protein was first discovered in brain, it is not specific to the nervous system. The quantity of brain is much higher than in the peripheral tissues, but it is present in heart, liver, and kidney.

How do these two α proteins, which are both pertussis toxin substrates, compare functionally? Both proteins have GTPase activity. The GTPase activity of the α_{39} protein is easily measured in solution (Neer et al. 1984). The GTPase activity of α_{41} is extremely low, unless it is reconstituted with a hormone receptor (Asano et al. 1984). Both α_{41} and α_{39} can couple to muscarinic cholinergic receptors in the brain as shown by Florio and Sternweis (1985).

The proteins differ in their affinity for $\beta \cdot \gamma$. One way to measure the affinity of α for $\beta \cdot \gamma$ is to make use of our observation that the isolated α subunit is not a substrate for ADP-ribosylation by pertussis toxin. The substrate is actually the $\alpha \cdot \beta \cdot \gamma$ heterotrimer. Therefore, we can measure the amount of $\beta \cdot \gamma$, which must be added to a fixed concentration of α_{41} or α_{39} in order to support ADP-ribosylation. This experiment, strictly speaking, measures a more complicated function than simply the affinity of α for $\beta \cdot \gamma$, but the clear result was that it takes about three times more $\beta \cdot \gamma$ to support ADP-ribosylation of α_{39} than to support ADP-ribosylation of α_{41} (Huff and Neer 1986). This may explain why α_{41} is a better substrate for ADP-ribosylation in membranes than α_{39}. In fact, depending on the stoichiometry of the two α subunits and $\beta \cdot \gamma$, it is possible that α_{39} would not be ADP-ribosylated at all. This is important to bear in mind when considering the guanine nucleotide-mediated hormonal effects that are not blocked by pertussis toxin (discussed below).

The overall conformation of the two proteins is extremely similar. This can be probed by looking at the peptides generated from the native protein by trypsin (Winslow et al. 1986). In the presence of GTPγS, both proteins lose a 2-kDa amino terminal fragment and generate stable 37-kDa and 39-kDa fragments, respectively. These fragments are not digested further by trypsin, even if they are incubated for a long time. In the absence of any stabilizing guanine nucleotide, both proteins are rapidly degraded to small fragments. The fragments generated in the presence of GTP are very different from the ones generated in the presence of a nonhydrolyzable GTP analogue. With GTP, the proteins pass quickly through the 37-kDa and 39-kDa forms and then are cleaved again to generate fragments of about 25 kDa and 17 kDa, which are stabilized by the GTP.

Susceptibility to proteolysis may also be used to determine whether ADP-ribosylation causes similar changes in the conformation of α_{41} and α_{39}. We found that it does not. Although the cleavage patterns of the two unribosylated proteins are similar, after modification the patterns are different. Since ADP-ribosylation induces distinct conformation in the two proteins, ADP-ribosylation might interfere more with the function of one protein than with the other (Winslow et al. 1986).

The biochemical studies suggesting that there is a multiplicity of guanine nucleotide-binding proteins are corroborated by genetic evidence. To generate more specific probes to study the α proteins and to determine how many α proteins actually exist, we set out to clone the α_{39} protein and related G proteins. We screened a bovine pituitary cDNA library at very low stringency using as a probe a full-length cDNA for transducin, which was kindly given to us by Dr. Melvin Simon of the California Institute of Technology. What we cloned out of this library was not, in fact, the highly abundant α_{39}, but α_{41}, and another cDNA encoding a putative GTP-binding protein, which, over the regions we sequenced, is 87% identical to α_{41}, (α_i).

We have called this cDNA pαh. It is clearly a separate gene from α_{41}, as shown by the analysis of genomic DNA by Southern hybridization (Michel et al. 1986).

This year has been the year of cloning the GTP-binding proteins, and the many laboratory groups have turned up an impressive array of different guanine nucleotide-binding proteins belonging both to the cholera toxin and to the pertussis toxin substrate family (Lochrie et al. 1985, Yatsunami and Khorana 1985, Itoh et al. 1986, Nukada et al. 1986a,b, Robishaw et al. 1986a,b, Sullivan et al. 1986, Michel et al. 1986). With so many α proteins identified, the task now is to determine which ones couple to which hormone receptors and to which output systems. This work is just beginning in our laboratory and in several others. One thing we can say is that at least one clonal line of cells, GH$_4$ pituitary cells, expresses both α_o and α_i. Thus, it seems that these different proteins are not segregated to different cell types, and a single cell must keep straight the coupling of a highly homologous family of proteins to a variety of effector molecules. Clearly, the availability of cDNA probes for these proteins will allow some extremely interesting experiments, both in terms of site-directed mutagenesis and of these proteins' expression in different cell lines.

FUNCTIONAL DOMAINS OF THE α PROTEINS

In the short run, the availability of deduced sequence information for these proteins allows us to design and interpret chemical experiments to define the functional domains of the α proteins. One approach to this problem is to introduce discrete chemical modifications into the protein and look at the functional consequences of these changes. We have taken this approach in studying the reactivity of the sulfhydryl groups in α_{39} (Winslow et al. 1987). In this protein, there are three sulfhydryls that can react with N-ethylmaleimide (NEM) in the unliganded α_{39}; only one is reactive in the presence of GTPγS. The GTPγS-insensitive sulfhydryl reacts more rapidly than the others, which makes it possible to create a singly substituted α_{39} module. Reaction of this GTPγS-insensitive, rapidly reactive sulfhydryl with NEM blocks the ADP-ribosylation of α_{39} by pertussis toxin. However, since the true substrate for pertussis toxin labeling is not α_{39}, but the α_{39} $\beta\cdot\gamma$ heterotrimer, reaction of this sulfhydryl might block ADP-ribosylation by preventing association of α_{39} with $\beta\cdot\gamma$. We showed by hydrodynamic measurements that this is not the case. When one sulfhydryl reacts, the $\alpha_{39}\cdot\beta\cdot\gamma$ heterotrimer still forms. To interpret these observations, we purified and sequenced the tryptic peptides containing the three reactive sulfhydryl groups. The biggest surprise was the rapidly reactive sulfhydryl. ADP-ribosylation of the G proteins is thought to occur on a cysteine residue 347, which is four amino acids from the carboxyl terminus (West et al. 1985). We had thought that this group would be the one to react rapidly with NEM. We found, however, that the rapidly reactive cysteine is at position 108, which is quite far in the linear sequence from the carboxyl terminus. Alkylation of this sulfhydryl may affect the reactivity of cys 347 either sterically or through an induced conformational change in α_{39}.

The closely related molecule transducin has a reaction pattern that is virtually identical to the one we observed in α_{39}. There are three reactive sulfhydryl groups in transducin, two sensitive to GTPγS and one insensitive (Ho and Fung 1984), although the sites of sulfhydryl modification have not yet been determined. However, the GTPγS-insensitive cysteine in a α_{39}, cys 108, is a cysteine that is not present at the position in transducin or any other α protein. Although the overall kinetics of NEM reaction with transducin and with α_{39} are superficially similar, the observation that at least one reactive residue must be different acts as a caution against a too-free generalization based on the striking structural and functional homology among the α subunits of G proteins.

Cloning the cDNAs encoding a variety of G proteins has made available the deduced amino acid sequences of the proteins. All G proteins known so far have in common four regions of homology to the GTP-binding oncogene product *ras* and to the GTP-binding bacterial protein, EFTu (elongation factor Tu) (Halliday 1984, Lochrie et al. 1985, Masters et al. 1986, Sullivan et al. 1986). The crystal structure of the guanine nucleotide-binding site of the latter protein was determined (Jurnak 1985, la Cour 1985) and the four homologous regions were shown to make up the active site of EFTu. This observation suggests that the regions of the G proteins which are homologous to EFTu also form the GTP-binding site. The homologous regions are shown as striped blocks in the diagram of α_{39} shown in Figure 10.3. The positions of the GTPγS-sensitive and insensitive sulfhydryls are indicated in the diagram. Neither of the GTPγS-sensitive sulfhydryls are within these regions thought to make up the GTP-binding site. We presume, therefore, that the effect of GTPγS on the sulfhydryl reactivity is the result of a conformational change in the molecule rather than direct steric hindrance, although this hypothesis still needs to be tested further.

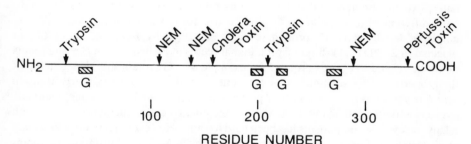

RESIDUE NUMBER

Figure 10.3. Structural and functional features of α_{39}. Sites of tryptic cleavage were identified by Hurley et al. (1984). The α_{39} has not yet been shown to be ADP-ribosylated by cholera toxin. However, the arginine, which is ADP-ribosylated by cholera toxin in transducin, is present in α_{39} (Itoh et al. 1986), and the sequences surrounding this residue are similar to those in transducin. Pertussis toxin has been shown to ADP-ribosylate residue 347 in transducin (West et al. 1985). The α_{39} protein contains the same cysteine and is highly homologous to transducin in this area (Itoh et al. 1986). The boxes marked G denote regions where α_{39} and other G proteins are homologous to *ras* protein and EFTu (Halliday 1984, Lochrie et al. 1985, Masters et al. 1986). These regions of EFTu make up the GTP-binding site (Jurnak 1985, laCour 1985). Because of the strong similarity of all the sequences, these sections are probably part of the genuine nucleotide binding regions of the G proteins. The cysteines modified by N-ethylmaleimide are at the arrows marked NEM. The reactivity of cysteine 108 is not affected by GTPγS; the other two sulfhydryls are blocked by GTPγS (Winslow et al. 1987).

Table 10.2. *Guanine Nucleotide-Dependent Hormone Actions Which are not Blocked by Pertussis Toxin*

Progesterone inhibition of adenylate cyclase in toad oocytes	Olate et al. (1984)
Carbachol stimulation of phosphodiesterase or phosphatidyl-inositide turnover in 1321N1 astrocytoma cells	Masters et al. (1985)
GTPγS-induced decrease of angiotensin II receptor affinity	Pobiner et al. (1985)
Thrombin-induced release of inositol and increased [86]Rb$^+$ uptake in 3T3 L1 fibroblasts	Murayama and Ui (1985)
TRH stimulation of phosphatidylinositol hydrolysis in GH$_3$ cells	Martin et al. (1986)
Angiotensin-stimulated prolactin release in anterior pituitary cells	Enjalbert et al. (1986)

Throughout this chapter, I have discussed the structure and function of G proteins of the $\alpha \cdot \beta \cdot \gamma$ type with highly homologous α and β subunits. Recent data suggest, however, that there may be other G proteins that do not fit this category. One line of evidence comes from the observation that some actions of guanine nucleotide-modulated receptors are neither coupled to α_s nor blocked by pertussis toxin. Table 10.2 shows some examples, although the list is not comprehensive. What G protein mediates these effects? One possibility is that it is α_{39} or an α_{39}-like protein since we have shown that α_{39} is not as good a substrate for ADP-ribosylation as α_{41}. An alternative explanation may be that these actions are mediated by G proteins with α subunits different from those in the G proteins that form $\alpha \cdot \beta \cdot \gamma$ heterotrimers. An example of the latter is the protein recently described by Evans et al. (1986) in placenta, a 21-kDa GTP-binding protein that seems to associate with $\beta \cdot \gamma$ and seems not to be related to the *ras* protein. An example of a G protein that shares many of the properties of the α subunits but seems not to associate with $\beta \cdot \gamma$ is *ras* itself. In *Saccharomyces cerevisiae*, the *ras* proteins are important in regulating adenylate cyclase activity (Katoaka et al. 1985). In mammalian cells, interaction of *ras* with adenylate cyclase components has been hard to show. However, a report by Wakelam et al. (1986) that expression of normal p21 N-*ras* in NIH 313 fibroblasts promotes the coupling of bombesin receptors to inositol phosphate production points to a possible role for *ras* in coupling hormone receptors to membrane-bound enzymes, which may be analogous to the role played by the classical G proteins. How useful this concept will be in defining the transforming function of *ras* remains to be seen.

The complexity of the G protein presents a formidable challenge. Not only must we determine the function of the many G proteins that have been described, but we must understand how the cell maintains the specificity of its responses when it contains so many extremely similar proteins. In vitro, the proteins can substitute for each other, and quite heterologous reconstitutions have been successful (for example, the β adrenergic receptor can couple to α_i [Asano et al. 1984, Kanaho et al.

1984, Cerione et al. 1985]). But cells have more rigorous requirements. The specificity in the cell might depend on the recognition of rather subtle differences among some of the G proteins. Or it is possible that receptors, G proteins and effectors are arranged in multiprotein complexes that do not exchange freely, except in unusual circumstances. The current problem is to define the mechanisms that allow the cell to activate specific, hormonally controlled pathways and to regulate differentially the function of individual receptors.

ACKNOWLEDGMENT

This work was supported by grant GM 36259 from the National Institutes of Health to the author.

REFERENCES

Asano T, Katada T, Gilman AG, Ross EM. 1984. Activation of the inhibitory GTP-binding protein of adenylate cyclase, G_i, by α-adrenergic receptors in reconstituted phospholipid vesicles. J Biol Chem 259:9351–9354.

Bender J, Wolf LG, Neer EJ. 1984. Interaction of forskolin with resolved adenylate cyclase components. Adv Cyclic Nucleotide Protein Phosphorylation Res 17:101–109.

Bokoch GM, Gilman AG. 1984. Inhibition of receptor-mediated release of arachidonic acid by pertussis toxin. Cell 39:301–308.

Brandt DR, Asano T, Pedersen SE, Ross EM. 1983. Reconstitution of catecholamine-stimulated guanosinetriphosphatase activity. Biochemistry 22:4357–4362.

Burch RM, Luini A, Axelrod J. 1986. Phospholipase A_2 and phospholipase C are activated by distinct GTP-binding proteins in response to α_1-adrenergic stimulation in FRTL5 thyroid cells. Proc Natl Acad Sci USA 83:7201–7205.

Cassel D, Pfeuffer T. 1978. Mechanism of cholera toxin action: Covalent modification of the guanyl nucleotide-binding protein of the adenylate cyclase system. Proc Natl Acad Sci USA 75:2669–2673.

Cassel D, Selinger Z. 1976. Catecholamine-stimulated GTPase activity in turkey erythrocyte membranes. Biochim Biophys Acta 452:538–551.

Cerione RA, Sibley DR, Codina J, et al. 1984. Reconstitution of a hormone-sensitive adenylate cyclase system. J Biol Chem 259:9979–9982.

Cerione RA, Staniszewski C, Benovic JL, Lefkowitz RJ, Caron MG. 1985. Specificity of the functional interactions of the β-adrenergic receptor and rhodopsin with guanine nucleotide regulatory proteins reconstituted in phospholipid vesicles. J Biol Chem 260:1493–1500.

Codina J, Hildebrandt J, Iyengar R, Birnbaumer L, Sekura RD, Manclark CR. 1983. Pertussis toxin substrate, the putative N_i component of adenylyl cyclases, is an $\alpha\beta$ heterodimer regulated by guanine nucleotide and magnesium. Proc Natl Acad Sci USA 80:4276–4280.

deLean A, Stadel J, Lefkowitz RJ. 1980. A ternary complex model explains the agonist-specific binding properties of the adenylate cyclase-coupled β-adrenergic receptor. J Biol Chem 255:7108–7117.

Enjalbert A, Sladeczek F, Guillon G, et al. 1986. Angiotensin II and dopamine modulate both cAMP and inositol phosphate productions in anterior pituitary cells. J Biol Chem 261:4071–4075.

Evans T, Brown ML, Fraser ED, Northup JK. 1986. Purification of the major GTP-binding proteins from human placental membranes. J Biol Chem 261:7052–7059.

Florio VA, Sternweis PC. 1985. Reconstitution of resolved muscarinic cholinergic receptors with purified GTP-binding proteins. J Biol Chem 260:3477–3483.

Fong HKW, Hurley JB, Hopkins RS, et al. 1986. Repetitive segmental structure of the trans-ducin β subunit: Homology with the CDC4 gene and identification of related mRNAs. Proc Natl Acad Sci USA 83:2162–2166.

Gill DM, Meren R. 1978. ADP-ribosylation of membrane proteins catalyzed by cholera toxin: Basis of the activation of adenylate cyclase. Proc Natl Acad Sci USA 75:3050–3054.

Halliday KR. 1984. Regional homology in GTP-binding proto-oncogene products and elongation factors. J Cyclic Nucleotide Protein Phosphor Res 9:435–448.

Harris BA, Robishaw JD, Mumby SM, Gilman AG. 1985. Molecular cloning of complemen-tary DNA for the alpha subunit of the G protein that stimulates adenylate cyclase. Science 229:1274–1277.

Hildebrandt JD, Birnbaumer L. 1983. Inhibitory regulation of adenylyl cyclase in the ab-sence of stimulatory regulation. Requirements and kinetics of guanine nucleotide-induced inhibition of the Cyc⁻ S49 adenylyl cyclase. J Biol Chem 258:13141–13147.

Hildebrandt JD, Codina J, Rosenthal W, et al. 1985. Characterization by two-dimensional peptide mapping of the α subunits of N_s and N_i, the regulatory proteins of adenylyl cyclase, and of transducin, the guanine nucleotide-binding protein of rod outer segments of the eye. J Biol Chem 260:14867–14872.

Ho YK, Fung BKK. 1984. Characterization of transducin from bovine retinal rod outer seg-ments. J Biol Chem 259:6694–6699.

Hoffman BB, Michel T, Brenneman TB, Lefkowitz RJ. 1982. Interactions of agonists with platelet α_2-adrenergic receptors. Endocrinology 110:926–932.

Huff RM, Axton JM, Neer EJ. 1985. Physical and immunological characterization of a guanine nucleotide-binding protein purified from bovine cerebral cortex. J Biol Chem 260:10864–10871.

Huff RM, Neer EJ. 1986. Subunit interactions of native and ADP-ribosylation α_{39} and α_{41}, two guanine nucleotide-binding proteins from bovine cerebral cortex. J Biol Chem 261:1105–1110.

Hurley JB, Simon MI, Teplow DB. 1984. Homologies between signal transducing G proteins and *ras* gene products. Science 226:860–862.

Itoh H, Kozasa T, Nagata S, et al. 1986. Molecular cloning and sequence determination of cDNAs for subunits of the guanine nucleotide-binding proteins G_s, G_i, and G_o from rat brain. Proc Natl Acad Sci USA 83:3776–3780.

Jurnak F. 1985. Structure of the GDP domain of EF-Tu and location of the amino acids ho-mologous to ras oncogene proteins. Science 230:32–36.

Kanaho Y, Tsai SC, Adamik R, Hewlett EL, Moss J, Vaughan M. 1984. Rhodopsin-enhanced GTPase activity of the inhibitory GTP-binding protein of adenylate cyclase. J Biol Chem 259:7378–7381.

Katada T, Northup JK, Bokoch GM, Ui M, Gilman AG. 1984. The inhibitory guanine nucleotide-binding regulatory component of adenylate cyclase. Subunit dissociation and guanine nucleotide-dependent hormonal inhibition. J Biol Chem 259:3578–3585.

Katada T, Ui M. 1982. Direct modification of the membrane adenylate cyclase system by islet-activating protein due to ADP-ribosylation of a membrane protein. Proc Natl Acad Sci USA 79:3129–3133.

Kataoka T, Powers S, Cameron S, et al. 1985. Functional homology of mammalian and yeast RAS genes. Cell 40:19–26.

la Cour TFM, Nyborg J, Thirup S, Clark BFC. 1985. Structural details of the binding of guanosine diphosphate to elongation factor Tu from E. coli as studied by X-ray crystallog-raphy. EMBO J 4:2385–2388.

Lefkowitz RJ, Caron MG, Michel T, Stadel J. 1982. Mechanisms of hormone receptor-effector coupling: the β-adrenergic receptor and adenylate cyclase. Fed Proc 41:2664–2670.

Lochrie MA, Hurley JB, Simon MI. 1985. Sequence of the alpha subunit of photoreceptor G protein: Homologies between transducin, ras, and elongation factors. Science 228:96–99.

Logothetis DE, Kurachi Y, Galper J, Neer EJ, Clapham DE. 1987. The βγ subunits of GTP-binding proteins activate the muscarinic K^+ channel in heart. Nature 325:321–326.

Londos C, Salomon Y, Lin MC, et al. 1974. 5'-guanylylimidodiphosphate, a potent activator of adenylate cyclase systems in eukaryotic cells. Proc Natl Acad Sci USA 71:3087–3090.

Martin TFJ, Lucas DO, Bajjalieh SM, Kowalchyk JA. 1986. Thyrotropin-releasing hormone activates a Ca^{2+}-dependent polyphosphoinositide phosphodiesterase in permeable GH_3 cells. J Biol Chem 261:2918–2927.

Masters SB, Martin MW, Harden TK, Brown JH. 1985. Pertussis toxin does not inhibit muscarinic-receptor-mediated phosphoinositide hydrolysis or calcium mobilization. Biochem J 227:933–937.

Masters SB, Stroud RM, Bourne HR. 1986. Family of G proteins α chains: Amphipathic analysis and predicted structure of functional domains. Protein Engineering 1:43–50.

Michel T, Winslow JW, Smith JA, Seidman JG, Neer EJ. 1986. Molecular cloning and characterization of cDNA encoding the GTP-binding protein α_i and identification of a related protein, α_h. Proc Natl Acad Sci USA 83:7663–7667.

Murayama T, Ui M. 1986. Receptor-mediated inhibition of adenylate cyclase and stimulation of arachidonic acid release in 3T3 fibroblasts. J Biol Chem 260:7226–7233.

Neer EJ, Lok JM, Wolf LG. 1984. Purification and properties of the inhibitory guanine nucleotide regulatory unit of brain adenylate cyclase. J Biol Chem 259:14222–14229.

Neer EJ, Wolf LG, Gill DM. 1987. The stimulatory guanine nucleotide regulatory unit of adenylate cyclase from bovine cerebral cortex: ADP-ribosylation and purification. Biochem J (in press).

Northup JK, Sternweis PC, Gilman AG. 1983a. The subunits of the stimulatory regulatory component of adenylate cyclase. Resolution, activity and properties of the 35,000 dalton protein. J Biol Chem 258:11361–11368.

Northup JK, Smigel MD, Sternweis PC, Gilman AG. 1983b. The subunits of the stimulatory regulatory component of adenylate cyclase. Resolution of the activated 45,000-dalton (α) subunit. J Biol Chem 258:11369–11376.

Nukada T, Tanabe T, Takahashi H, et al. 1986a. Primary structure of the α-subunit of bovine adenylate cyclase-stimulating G-protein deduced from the cDNA sequence. FEBS Lett 195:220–224.

Nukada T, Tanabe T, Takahashi H, et al. 1986b. Primary structure of the α-subunit of bovine adenylate cyclase-inhibiting G-protein deduced from the cDNA sequence. FEBS Lett 197:305–310.

Olate J, Allende CC, Allende JE, Sekura RD, Birmbaumer L. 1984. Oocyte adenylyl cyclase contains N_i, yet the guanine nucleotide-dependent inhibition by progresterone is not sensitive to pertussis toxin. FEBS Lett 175:25.

Pederson SE, Ross EM. 1982. Functional reconstitution of β-adrenergic receptors and the stimulatory GTP-binding protein of adenylate cyclase. Proc Natl Acad Sci USA 79:7228–7232.

Pobiner BF, Hewlett EL, Garrison JC. 1985. Role of N_i in coupling angiotensin receptors to inhibition of adenylate cyclase in hepatocytes. J Biol Chem 260:16200–16209.

Robishaw JD, Russell DW, Harris BA, Smigel MD, Gilman AG. 1986a. Deduced primary structure of the α subunit of the GTP-binding stimulatory protein of adenylate cyclase. Proc Natl Acad Sci USA 83:1251–1255.

Robishaw JD, Smigel MD, Gilman AG. 1986b. Molecular basis for two forms of the G protein that stimulates adenylate cyclase. J Biol Chem 261:9587–9590.

Smigel M, Katada T, Northup JK, Bokoch GM, Ui M, Gilman AG. 1984. Mechanisms of guanine nucleotide-mediated regulation of adenylate cyclase activity. Adv Cyclic Nucleotide Protein Phosphorylation Res 17:1–18.

Steer ML, Wood A. 1979. Regulation of human platelet adenylate cyclase by epinephrine, prostaglandin E_1, and guanine nucleotides. J Biol Chem 254:10791–10797.

Sternweis PC. 1986. The purified α subunits of G_o and G_i from bovine brain require βγ for association with phospholipid vesicles. J Biol Chem 261:631–637.

Sternweis PC, Robishaw JD. 1984. Isolation of two proteins with high affinity for guanine nucleotides from membranes of bovine brain. J Biol Chem 259:13806–13813.

Sullivan KA, Liao YC, Alborzi A, et al. 1986. Inhibitory and stimulatory G proteins of adenylate cyclase: cDNA and amino acid sequences of the chains. Proc Natl Acad Sci USA 83:6687–6691.

Sunyer T, Codina J, Birnbaumer L. 1984. GTP hydrolysis by pure N_i, the inhibitory regulatory component of adenylyl cyclases. J Biol Chem 259:15447–15451.

Tolkovsky AM, Braun S, Levitzki A. 1982. Kinetics of interaction between the β-receptor, the GTP regulatory protein, and the catalytic unit of turkey erythrocyte adenylate cyclase. Proc Natl Acad Sci USA 79:213–217.

Tsai SC, Adamik R, Kanaho Y, Hewlett EL, Moss J. 1984. Effects of guanyl nucleotides and rhodopsin on ADP-ribosylation of the inhibitory GTP-binding component of adenylate cyclase by pertussis toxin. J Biol Chem 259:15320–15323.

Ui M, Katada T, Murayama T, et al. 1984. Islet-activating protein, pertussis toxin: a specific uncoupler of receptor-mediated inhibition of adenylate cyclase. Adv Cyclic Nucleotide Res 17:145–152.

Van Dop C, Tsubokawa M, Bourne HR, Ramachandran J. 1984a. Amino acid sequence of retinal transducin at the site ADP-ribosylated by cholera toxin. J Biol Chem 259:696–698.

Van Dop C, Yamanaka G, Steinberg F, et al. 1984b. ADP-ribosylation of transducin by pertussis toxin blocks the light-stimulated hydrolysis of GTP and cGMP in retinal photoreceptors. J Biol Chem 259:23–26.

Wakelam MJO, Davies SA, Houslay MD, McKay I, Marshall CJ, Hall A. 1986. Normal p21[N-ras] couples bombesin and other growth factor receptors to inositol phosphate production. Nature 323:173–176.

West RE, Moss J, Vaughan M, Liu T, Liu TY. 1985. Pertussis toxin-catalyzed ADP-ribosylation of transducin. J Biol Chem 260:14428–14430.

Winslow JW, Bradley JD, Smith JA, Neer EJ. 1987. Reactive sulfhydryl groups of α_{39}, a guanine nucleotide-binding protein from brain: Location and function. J Biol Chem 262:4501–4507.

Winslow JW, Van Amsterdam JR, Neer EJ. 1986. Conformations of the α_{39}, α_{41}, and $\beta\cdot\gamma$ components of brain guanine nucleotide-binding proteins. J Biol Chem 261:7571–7579.

Yatsunami K, Khorana HG. 1985. GTPase of bovine rod outer segments: The amino acid sequence of the α subunit as derived from the cDNA sequence. Proc Natl Acad Sci USA 82:4316–4320.

Symposium on Fundamental Cancer Research, Vol. 39.
© 1987 by The University of Texas System Cancer Center.

11. Genetic and Biochemical Analysis of *ras* p21 Structure

Frank McCormick, Corey Levenson,* Georgette Cole,*
Michael Innis,[†] and Robin Clark

*Departments of Molecular Biology, *Chemistry, and [†]Microbial Genetics,
Cetus Corporation, Emeryville, California 94608*

We tested aspects of our model of the *ras* p21 structure using generic, biochemical, and immunologic approaches. First, we made a monoclonal antibody against a p21 region that is highly conserved and likely to be critical to p21 function. The antibody blocks p21 function in various cell systems. Its binding to p21 is completely blocked by guanine nucleotides, even though the region of p21 to which it binds does not seem to be part of the guanine nucleotide-binding site. We propose that the conformation of this critical region is modulated by nucleotide binding. Another interesting region of p21 includes amino acids 116 and 119, which seem to confer, in part, the specificity of p21 for guanine nucleotides. We made a series of mutants in this region and tested their ability to bind GTP, and such related purine nucleotides as XTP and diaminopurine nucleoside triphosphate. We were able to refine our model for guanine nucleotide interaction with p21 and to create mutant proteins with altered specificity for purine nucleotides.

Finally, we tested rates of autophosphorylation of six position 12 mutants and conclude that amino acid 12 affects the positioning of bound nucleotides relative to sequences around amino acid 59.

We have previously developed a model for the tertiary structure of the p21, the product of the *ras* family of proto-oncogenes and oncogenes (McCormick et al. 1985). Here we report the further development of this model, using in vitro mutagenesis and biochemical analysis to test and refine several aspects. Figure 11.1 shows the proposed structure of the highly conserved region of *ras* gene products, including the p21 proteins encoded by mammalian cells and the *ras* gene products of *Saccaromyces cerivisae* and *S. pombei* and of *Drosophila* and *Aplysia*. In this chapter, we will focus on three regions of the proposed structure: the phosphoryl binding region, which includes the GTPase site, the guanine specificity region, and the region proposed to interact with an unidentified cellular component in a guanine nucleotide-dependent fashion (region 30–50).

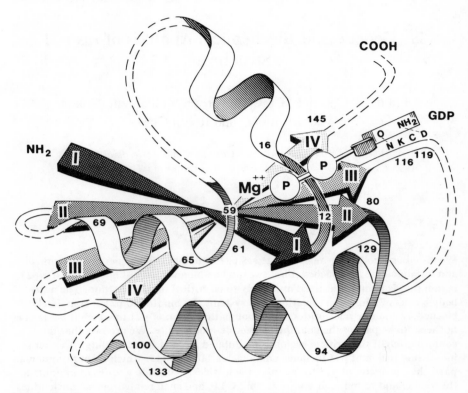

Figure 11.1. Proposed structure of the highly conserved region of *ras* gene products.

THE PHOSPHORYL BINDING REGION

The phosphoryl binding region appears to be composed of two regions comprising amino acids 12–15 and 57–63. The first of these regions contains the glycine residues 12 and 13, replacement of which by other amino acids results in activation of the p21 protein. These replacements also affect the GTPase activity of the protein, as described by others (Sweet et al. 1984, McGrath et al. 1984, Gibbs et al. 1984, Manne et al. 1985, Der et al. 1986). We have compared the GTPase activity and guanine nucleotide–binding properties of human N-*ras* p21 with glycine, aspartate or valine at position 12 and have found the two mutant forms retain 40% and 12% of wild-type activities, but do not differ significantly in their affinities for GTP or GDP (Trahey et al. 1987). These results are consistent with the notion that reduction of GTPase activity brings about activation of p21 by reducing the rate of conversion of bound GTP to GDP. However, as others have noted, there is no correlation between alteration in GTPase activity and transforming potential as would be expected from such a model.

By analogy with bacterial elongation factor Tu (EFTu), and from direct bio-chemical analysis (Tucker et al. 1986), it appears that the oxygen atoms of alpha and beta phosphates of bound GDP interact directly with the 12–15 region of p21. One of these interactions may include the amino group of Lys-15 (Sigal et al. 1986), and the others may be interactions with main chain residues. We have argued else-where (McCormick et al. 1985) that mutations at glycine-12 affect GTPase activity by changing the conformation of the flexible 12–15 loop; glycine is unique in allowing a wide range of main-chain dihedral angles that are not possible with amino acids with side chains. Proline is exceptional in allowing a main-chain di-hedral angle not possible with other amino acids, except, of course, glycine. This may account for the observation that replacement of glycine with proline does not affect transforming activity or GTPase activity of p21. We may therefore speculate that the exact positioning of phosphoryl groups of guanine nucleotides in the bind-ing sites depends on specific interactions in the 12–15 region and on conformations of the main chain determined in part by the presence of glycine at position 12.

The p21 proteins encoded by Harvey sarcoma virus and Kirsten sarcoma virus contain mutations at position 59 (threonine instead of alanine) that are substrates for autophosphorylation: the gamma phosphate of bound GTP is transferred to the side chain hydroxyl moiety. This reaction shows that the 57–63 region is close to the 12–15 region in the binding site (Fig. 11.1). We have made several mutations at position 12 in viral K-*ras* p21 and determined how these mutations affect auto-phosphorylation. Table 11.1 shows that all of the mutations, except aspartate-12, increase the rate of autophosphorylation relative to the glycine-12 form. These al-tered rates may reflect slightly different orientations of the phosphate groups of bound GTP relative to threonine-59. Replacement of threonine-59 with serine-59 resulted in a fourfold drop in rate of autophosphorylation. This could be because

Table 11.1. *p21 Autophosphorylation*

Position 12 Substitution	Relative Activity
Gly	1.0
Ser	3.7
Val	1.5
Arg	2.5
Asp	0.24
Ala	1.7
Cys	1.3

Aliquots of *E. coli* extracts containing v-Ki-*ras* p21 with indicated substitutions at position 12 were immunoprecipitated with monoclonal antibody Y13-259 and washed immune complexes were resuspended in autophosphorylation buffer (100 mM NaCl, 2 mM $MgCl_2$, 20 mM Tris pH 8.0, 0.1% NP_4O, 1 mM DTT) for 3 hr at 37°C in the presence of 5 μ Ciγ-^{32}P-GTP. After washing, p21 was eluted and separated by sodium dodecyl sulfate polyacrylamide gel electrophoresis and visualized by autoradiography. Autophosphorylation was quantitated by densitometry. Relative amounts of p21 in the seven extracts were determined by immunoblotting using a monoclonal antibody that reacts with all forms of p21 as a probe and p21 levels were determined, as above, by densitometry. Autophosphorylation activity is expressed relative to the glycine substitution (1 unit) after normalizing for p21 content.

the methyl group of threonine renders the hydroxyl group slightly more nucleo-
phylic than the hydroxyl group of serine or because of favorable steric constraints
imposed by the methyl group.

It has been proposed that a magnesium ion forms a salt bridge between the two
phosphoryl binding regions, connecting aspartate-57 to the phosphoryl groups of
bound guanine nucleotide (Jurnak 1985). A mutant form of p21 that contains
alanine-57 instead of aspartate-57 does not bind GTP in vitro (data not shown), con-
firming the involvement of aspartate-57 in nucleotide binding. The magnesium ion
is also likely to be involved in hydrolysis of bound GTP, although it is not yet known
whether an additional magnesium ion may serve this function. In any event, the salt
bridge between bound nucleotide and aspartate-57 may be critical to p21 function.
The dimensions of this bridge are almost certainly different for p21.GDP and
p21.GTP, which raises the possibility that the positioning of the 57–63 loop relative
to the 12–15 loop varies with the state of phosphorylation of the bound nucleotide.

THE PUTATIVE EFFECTOR-BINDING REGION

The proposal that sequences between the two phosphoryl binding regions interact
with a cellular component in a guanine nucleotide–dependent manner is based on the
four following arguments. First, the equivalent region of EFTu interacts with aminoacyl-tRNA with an affinity that is three orders of magnitude higher for EFTu.GTP
than EFTu.GDP (Weissbach 1979). Hydrolysis of bound GTP by EFTu on ribosomes thus reduces the affinity for aminoacyl-tRNA, allowing dissociation and release of EFTu.GDP. This binary complex then exchanges bound GDP for GTP in
the presence of a protein referred to as EFTs and rebinds aminoacyl-tRNA. Direct
analysis of EFTu.GDP and EFTu.GTP structure has revealed that these complexes
do indeed exist in different conformations (Weissbach 1979). Second, a monoclonal
antibody raised against amino acids 29–44 neutralizes p21 function in various biological systems. Third, binding of this monoclonal to p21 is inhibited by GTP and
GDP but not by ATP or other nonbinding nucleotides. This suggests that GDP and
GTP maintain the 29–44 region in a conformation unsuitable for antibody binding.
In the absence of nucleotide, the protein appears to adopt a different conformation
in this region. Fourth, specific point mutations in this region inactivate p21 function
without affecting the guanine nucleotide–binding properties of p21.

GUANINE SPECIFICITY REGION

By analogy with the GDP-binding region of EFTu (McCormick et al. 1985, Jurnak
1985), it appears likely that asparagine-116 and aspartate-119 interact with bound
nucleotide in such a way as to confer specificity for guanine. We, and others, have
made mutant p21s that contain substitutions at these positions (Sigal et al. 1986),
and these mutations result in decreased affinity for guanine nucleotides. We have
also sought to change the specificity of p21 for guanine nucleotides by replacing
asparagine-116 with aspartate-116, or by replacing aspartate-119 with asparagine-

Table 11.2. *Nucleotide-Binding Properties of Position 116 and 119 Mutants*

Amino Acid		GTP	DAPTP	XTP	ATP
116	119				
Asn	Asp	+	−	+	−
Ala	Asp	−	−	ND	−
Asp	Asp	−	−	ND	−
Asp	Ala	−	ND	ND	−
Asn	Ala	−	ND	−	−
Asn	Asn	−	ND	+	−

Filter-binding assays were performed as described by McGrath et al. 1984.
+—detectable binding; −—no detectable binding; ND—not done.

119 (Table 11.2). In the first case, we expected the mutant to bind diaminopurine nucleoside diphosphate; this purine nucleotide contains an amino side group instead of the carbonyl group of guanine. However, this nucleotide did not bind to the mutant p21 or to wild-type p21. Furthermore, the aspartate-116 mutant did not bind GDP. These data suggest that the interaction between the side chain of amino acid 116 and the side group of guanine is not a simple hydrogen bond and that the carbonyl group of guanine interacts with additional amino acids, possibly from the other face of the nucleotide-binding pocket. Replacing aspartate-119 with asparagine resulted in a p21 protein that binds XTP (xanthosine diphosphate) but not GTP. We introduced this mutation into Harvey sarcoma virus p21 and observed that the transforming potential of the altered viral p21 was not reduced. Similar results have been reported elsewhere (Feig et al. 1986). This suggests that a complex between asparagine-119 p21 and XTP may be active in transformation. This altered specificity suggests that the 119 side chain does interact with the side group of the bound purine in a manner that imparts specificity. To our surprise, wild-type p21 also bound XTP. This observation implies that aspartate-119 is uncharged in the binding pocket, so that it can act as a hydrogen bond acceptor or donor, depending on the bound nucleotide.

SUMMARY

We have used the technique of site-directed mutagenesis to test various aspects of a model for p21 tertiary structure. From these experiments we conclude that asparate-57 is necessary for nucleotide binding, and it probably forms a salt bridge with magnesium. This salt bridge connects two regions of the phosphoryl binding site and may determine the conformation of the effector region of p21. We also conclude that the positioning of bound nucleotide relative to the 57–63 region is determined in part by the amino acid at position 12, and that amino acids 116 and 119 are involved in GTP binding. Amino acid 119 (aspartate) appears to interact directly with amino side group of guanine and is partly responsible for the specificity of p21 for GTP and XTP.

ACKNOWLEDGMENT

We thank Lauri Goda and Dragan Spasic for technical assistance.

REFERENCES

Der CJ, Finkel T, Cooper GM. 1986. Biological and biochemical properties of human *ras*H genes mutated at codon 61. Cell 44:167–176.

Feig LA, Pan B-T, Roberts TM, Cooper GM. 1986. Isolation of *ras* GTP-binding mutants using an in-situ colony-binding assay. Proc Natl Acad Sci USA 83:4607–4611.

Gibbs JB, Sigal IS, Poe M, Scolnick EM. 1984. Intrinsic GTPase activity distinguishes normal and oncogenic *ras* p21 molecules. Proc Natl Acad Sci USA 81:5704–5708.

Jurnak F. 1985. Structure of the GDP domain of EF-Tu and location of the amino acids homologous to *ras* oncogene proteins. Science 230:32–36.

Manne V, Bekesi E, Kung HF. 1985. Ha-*ras* proteins exhibit GTPase activity: Point mutations that activate Ha-*ras* gene products result in decreased GTPase activity. Proc Natl Acad Sci USA 82:376–380.

McCormick F, Clark BF, la Cour TF, Kjeldgaard M, Norskov-Lauritsen L, Nyborg J. 1985. A model for the tertiary structure of p21, the product of the *ras* oncogene. Science 230:78–82.

McGrath JP, Capon DJ, Goeddel DV, Levinson AD. 1984. Comparative biochemical properties of normal and activated human *ras* p21 protein. Nature 310:644–649.

Sigal IS, Gibbs JB, D'Alonzo JS, et al. 1986. Mutant *ras*-encoded proteins with altered nucleotide binding exert dominant biological effects. Proc Natl Acad Sci USA 83:952–956.

Sweet RW, Yokoyama S, Kamata T, Feramisco JR, Rosenberg M, Gross M. 1984. The product of *ras* is a GTPase and the T24 oncogenic mutant is deficient in this activity. Nature 311:273–275.

Trahey M, Milley RJ, Cole GE, et al. 1987. Biochemical and biological properties of human N-*ras* p21 protein. Mol Cell Biol 7:541–544.

Tucker J, Sczakiel G, Feuerstein J, John J, Goody RS, Wittinghofer A. 1986. Expression of p21 proteins in *E. coli* and stereochemisty of the nucleotide binding site. EMBO J 5:1351–1358.

Weissbach H. 1979. Soluble factors in protein synthesis. *In* Chamblis G, Craven C, Davies J, et al., eds., Ribosomes: Structure, Function and Genetics. University Park Press, Baltimore, pp. 377–441.

INTRACELLULAR SIGNALING

INTRODUCTION TO PART FIVE

Symposium on Fundamental Cancer Research, Vol. 39.

12. Mechanism of Regulation of Protein Kinase C by Lipid Second Messengers

Robert M. Bell, Yusuf A. Hannun,* and Carson R. Loomis

*Departments of Biochemistry and * Medicine, Duke University Medical Center, Durham, North Carolina 27710*

Protein kinase C (PKC), a Ca^{2+}- and phospholipid-dependent protein kinase, is now known to be regulated by sn-1,2-diacylglycerol (DAG) second messengers and is the intracellular phorbol ester receptor. Models of transmembrane signaling events that elicit DAG production include receptor-mediated G protein-dependent activation of phospholipase C. Several products of oncogenes resemble transmembrane signaling elements; critical second-messenger levels may, therefore, be altered by genetic defects in these elements. We found that normal rat kidney cells transformed with ras and sis contained elevated levels of DAG, and cells transformed with temperature-sensitive K-ras had elevated DAG levels at the permissive but not the restrictive temperature.

To study the mechanism of PKC activation by phosphatidylserine (PS), DAG, and Ca^{2+}, we used mixed micelles of Triton X-100, and analogous methods to examine PS dependence on [^{3}H]phorbol-dibutyrate binding and activation. PKC activation occurs at physiological mole fractions of PS and DAG and does not require a bilayer. Activation by PS, which was cooperative, required four or more molecules. Activation by DAG was not cooperative and one molecule was sufficient. Monomeric PKC is the active species. Our activation model suggests that PKC binds to Ca^{2+} and four PS carboxyl groups to form a surface-bound, "primed" but inactive complex. DAG binds to the complex of the four PS carboxyl groups, the Ca^{2+}, and the PKC through three bonds, two to ester carbonyls and one to the 3-hydroxyl moiety. Collectively, these may cause a conformational change and activate the enzyme.

The Ca^{2+}- and phospholipid-dependent protein kinase C, an intracellular receptor of phorbol ester tumor promoters, is regulated by sn-1,2-diacylglycerol (DAG) and Ca^{2+} second messengers (Nishizuka 1984). Protein kinase C plays a central role in intracellular transduction of extracellular signals, including neurotransmitters, growth factors, and hormones (Nishizuka 1983, 1984, Berridge 1984). This mechanism of transmembrane signaling involves receptor-mediated degradation of phosphatidylinositol 4,5 bisphosphate (PIP$_2$) to produce two second messengers, DAG and IP$_3$ (Fig. 12.1). IP$_3$ is believed to function in the mobilization of intracellular calcium (Berridge 1984), whereas DAG activates protein kinase C. Models of trans-

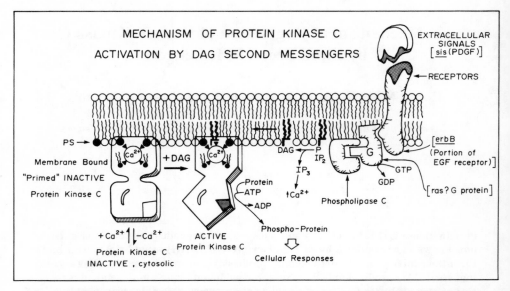

Figure 12.1. Model of transmembrane signaling and protein kinase C activation by diacylglycerol second messengers. (Reproduced from Bell 1986, with permission of *Cell.*)

membrane signaling depict a receptor-mediated G protein (GTP)–dependent activation of phospholipase C.

Interest is focused on protein kinase C because it is the target of tumor promoters and because several oncogene products resemble elements known to be involved in transmembrane signaling (Fig. 12.1). Alteration of critical second messenger levels may, therefore, occur as a result of genetic defects in these elements. The hypothesis that the DAGs produced in response to growth factors stimulate cell proliferation is supported by studies using cell-permeable DAGs (Nishizuka 1984, Davis et al. 1985, Rozengurt et al. 1984, Ganong et al. 1986a review).

QUANTITATIVE MEASUREMENTS OF DAG LEVELS IN *RAS* AND *SIS*-TRANSFORMED CELLS

In order to test whether specific oncogenes alter the levels of DAG second messengers, we developed a sensitive assay for the quantitation of DAG mass present in crude lipid extracts of cells by extension of the work of Kennerly et al. (1979). The assay employed *Escherichia coli* DAG kinase, overproduced in a plasmid-bearing strain to about 15% of the membrane protein (Loomis et al. 1985) and defined mixed micellar conditions (Walsh and Bell 1986) to solubilize the DAG present in crude lipid extracts and allow its quantitative conversion to [^{32}P]phosphatidic acid (Preiss et al. 1986). The assay was linear over the range of 25 pmol to 25 nmol. When we used this assay, levels of DAG in platelets and hepatocytes increased 210% and 230% over basal levels in response to thrombin and vasopressin, respectively, and when others have used other methods (most frequently radiolabeling), similar elevations of DAG in response to extracellular agents have been observed in numerous cell types. The amount of DAG present in normal rat kidney (NRK) cells grown at 34° and 38°C were 0.47 and 0.61 nmol/100 nmol of phospholipid, respectively. The amount of DAG increased 168% and 138% in K-*ras*-transformed NRK cells grown at 34°C and 38°C, respectively. When a temperature-sensitive K-*ras*-transformed NRK cell line was investigated, the amount of DAG was not elevated at the restrictive temperature but was elevated at the permissive temperature. The data are consistent with the K-*ras* gene product's functioning in transmembrane signaling by activating a phospholipase C. These mass measurements extend the work of Fleishmann et al. (1986) on DAG levels in *ras*-transformed cells. Elevated levels of DAG were also seen in *sis*-transformed NRK cells (Preiss et al. 1986). The data support the hypothesis that altered levels of DAG second messengers and protein kinase C activation (Anderson 1985) play important roles in cellular transformation. The methods developed should allow critical tests of the effects of other oncogenes on the mass of DAG in transformed cells.

STOICHIOMETRY OF PHOSPHOLIPID AND DAG COFACTOR REQUIREMENTS FOR PROTEIN KINASE C ACTIVATION

Protein kinase C activity, discovered in rat brain cytosol, was initially shown to be dependent on Ca^{2+} and phospholipids (Nishizuka 1984). The activation of protein kinase C involves translocation of the enzyme to the surface of the phospholipid vesicles (membranes) in a Ca^{2+}-dependent process. Phospholipid composition markedly affected activity; phosphatidylserine (PS) was most effective. That DAG is an activator of protein kinase C was discovered later, when it was shown that DAG increased the affinity of the enzyme for PS and for Ca^{2+} (Kishimoto 1980). The purified enzyme from rat brain has an apparent molecular weight of 80,000 (Nishizuka 1984).

The physical properties of sonic dispersions of phospholipids and diacylglycerols/phorbol esters have hampered efforts to determine the number of phospholipid and DAG molecules required for activation and efforts to define precisely the specificity of the phospholipid and DAG requirements. To circumvent these problems, investigators in our laboratory developed a mixed micellar assay for protein kinase C (Hannun et al. 1985). This method permits the number of DAG and PS molecules present in Triton X-100 mixed micelles to be independently and systematically varied. At 8 mol% PS in the presence of Ca^{2+}, activity was strongly dependent on *sn*-1,2-dioleoylglycerol ($diC_{18:1}$); maximal activity was observed at 1 mol% $diC_{18:1}$ (Fig. 12.2A). At this point, an average of 1.4 molecules of $diC_{18:1}$ would be present per mixed micelle. Since activation occurred at levels substantially below 1 mol%, the data imply that a single molecule of $diC_{18:1}$ is sufficient to activate protein kinase C. At 12 mol% PS, maximum activity was observed at 0.1 mol% $diC_{18:1}$ (Fig. 12.2C), where only one micelle in seven would have a single molecule of $diC_{18:1}$. Plasma membranes contain 8-20 mol% PS. Activation in mixed micelles establishes that a phospholipid bilayer is not required.

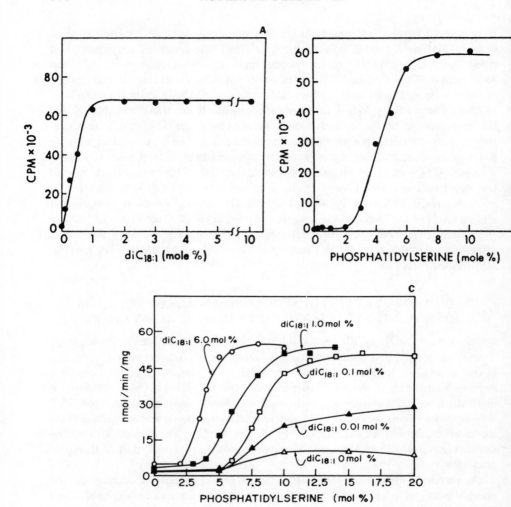

Figure 12.2. A. Diacylglycerol dependence of protein kinase C activation by mixed micelles. Mixed micelles were formed with 8.0 mol% PS. One mol% of $diC_{18:1}$ corresponds to $43\mu M$. $CaCl_2$ was added to a final concentration of 100 μM. (Reproduced from Hannun et al. 1985, with permission of *J Biol Chem*.) **B.** Phosphatidylserine dependence of protein kinase C activation by mixed micelles. $DiC_{18:1}$ was present at 2.5 mol% (107 μM) and $CaCl_2$ at 100 μM. One mole percent PS corresponds to 43 μM. (Reproduced from Hannun et al. 1985, with permission of *J Biol Chem*.) **C.** Phosphatidylserine and diacylglycerol interdependence of protein kinase C activation by mixed micelles. Activity measured in the absence of $diC_{18:1}$ △) and in the presence of $diC_{18:1}$ at 0.01 (▲), 0.1 (□), 1.0 (■), and 6.0 mol% (○). $CaCl_2$ was present at 100 μM. (Reproduced from Hannun et al. 1986a with permission of *J Biol Chem*.)

At 2.5 mol% $diC_{18:1}$, the activation of protein kinase C by PS was cooperative (Fig. 12.2B). A Hill number of 4.8 was calculated from these data, whereas a Hill number of 1 was calculated from the $diC_{18:1}$ dependence (Fig. 12.2A). Since protein kinase C activity begins to increase at 3 mol% PS, these data imply that four molecules of PS are the minimum number required for activation. Molecular sieve chromatography of protein kinase C, Triton X-100 mixed micelles containing PS and of the protein kinase C–mixed micellar complex indicated that monomeric (80 kDa) protein kinase C was the active species (Hannun et al. 1985). Protein kinase C binding to mixed micelles was dependent on PS and Ca^{2+} but not on DAG. As shown in Figure 12.2C (Hannun et al. 1986a), the activation of protein kinase C by PS and $diC_{18:1}$ proved to be interdependent. These data further support the implied stoichiometry of four PS molecules and one DAG being required for activation.

The mixed micelle methods have been extended to investigate the PS dependence of the activation of protein kinase C by phorbol esters and the PS dependence of [³H]phorbol-dibutyrate binding to protein kinase C (Hannun and Bell 1986). Monomeric protein kinase C is the species capable of binding phorbol esters and being activated by them (Hannun and Bell 1986). These data imply a similar mechanism of protein kinase C activation by DAG and phorbol esters and further support a stoichiometry of monomeric protein kinase C-4 $PS-Ca^{2+}-DAG$ (phorbol ester).

STRUCTURAL FEATURES OF DIACYLGLYCEROLS REQUIRED FOR PROTEIN KINASE C ACTIVATION

When the chain length of fatty acids present in DAG was systematically varied, protein kinase C was activated by all those DAGs of sufficient hydrophobic character that they were expected to partition into phospholipid vesicles or mixed micelles (Ganong et al. 1986a). Thus, sn-1,2-dioctanoylglycerol (diC_8) was as effective at activating protein kinase C in vitro as was $diC_{18:1}$ or 1-stearoyl-2-arachidonylglycerol (most prominent molecular species derived from PI) (Hannun et al. 1986a). Fatty-acid chain length was not important nor was the presence of unsaturated fatty acids required (Ganong et al. 1986b). However, sn-1,2-dibutyroylglycerol, which is very soluble and lacks significant hydrophobic character, was not effective in activating protein kinase C in vitro or in cells. DAGs containing long-chain fatty acids have limited water solubility and have proved to be difficult to deliver to cells. On the other hand, diC_8 has proved to be cell permeable and able to activate protein kinase C effectively in numerous cell types (Ganong et al. 1986a).

A series of more than 20 DAG analogues were prepared and tested as activators and antagonists of protein kinase C to determine the exact structural features required for activation (Ganong et al. 1985b). These analogues focused on the structural features present at the polar portion of the molecule, which would be expected to reside at the membrane interface where protein kinase C interacts. In brief, these analogues established that the sn-3-hydroxyl moiety was essential, that the position of the sn-3-hydroxyl was critical, that both oxygen esters are required (ethers and amides were inactive) (Ganong et al. 1986b), and that activation was stereospecific

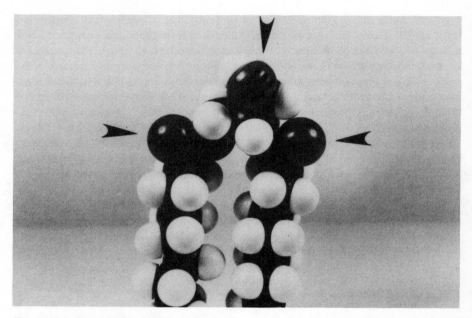

Figure 12.3. Space-filling model of *sn*-1,2-diacylglycerol. The photograph is of the molecule oriented in a phospholipid bilayer such that the hydroxyl and carbonyls are present at the interface. The arrows indicate the three positions thought to form crucial contacts with the protein kinase C-Ca^{2+}-PS complex responsible for activation: the 3′ hydroxyl oxygen and the two carbonyl oxygens of the ester bonds. (Figure 5 of Ganong et al. 1986b.)

(Hannun et al. 1986a, Boni and Rando 1985). The three functional groups (Fig. 12.3), *sn*-3-hydroxyl and 2-carbonyls of oxygen esters, were thought to form three bonds to the protein kinase C-4 PS-Ca^{2+} complex during activation (Fig. 12.4) (Ganong et al. 1986b).

MODEL OF PROTEIN KINASE C ACTIVATION BY PS, DAG, AND CA^{2+}

A model consistent with the available data was formulated (Ganong et al. 1986b). Four molecules of PS on the surface of a membrane (or micelle) are envisioned to bind Ca^{2+} through their carboxyl groups (Fig. 12.4). Such a complex would be analogous to that seen in EDTA or EGTA or that occurring in calmodulin. Protein kinase C is envisioned to bind to the 4 PS-Ca^{2+} complex (Fig. 12.4) and thereby become membrane bound, "primed," but inactive (Fig. 12.1). DAG (phorbol ester) is envisioned to bind to the 4 PS-Ca^{2+}-protein kinase C complex by occupying the position beneath the Ca^{2+} coordination sphere such that a direct bond between DAG and Ca^{2+} forms along with two other bonds between DAG and protein kinase C itself (Fig. 12.4D and E). This model accounts for the observed phospholipid dependencies, the increased affinity of protein kinase C for both PS and Ca^{2+} caused by DAG, and results with a photoactivable phorbol ester, in which lipids rather than enzyme were predominantly labeled (Delclos et al. 1983). The available data suggest a common mechanism of DAG and phorbol ester activation of protein kinase C; additional bonds are postulated between phorbol esters and protein kinase C to account for the higher affinity of phorbol esters. The model, while consistent with available data, is speculative; hopefully, it will be useful in the design of experiments furthering the understanding of the molecular mechanism of protein kinase regulation (Ganong et al. 1986).

MIXED MICELLE METHODS OF ANALYSIS OF PROTEIN KINASE C INHIBITORS

Interpretation of studies of putative specific inhibitors of protein kinase C is fraught with difficulties because these agents are amphipathic. Since the mixed micellar methods developed for protein kinase C permit the number of lipid cofactors per micelle to be systematically and independently varied, the approach can be readily extended to amphipathic inhibitors. The phenothiazine inhibitors of protein kinase C exerted their effects at a mole percent similar to the mole percent PS required for activation, which implied stoichiometric interactions (Hannun YA and Bell RM, unpublished data). The implied mechanism involved disruption of DAG/phorbol ester interaction with protein kinase C. It is important to note that the surface activity of the inhibitors is easily demonstrated because protein kinase C activity is independent of micelle number. Thus, when the number of mixed micelles containing a fixed mole percent PS and DAG are increased, the inhibitory powers of amphipathic surface-active inhibitors is lessened; inhibition, like activation, is then a function of the mole percent rather than the bulk concentration.

INHIBITION OF PROTEIN KINASE C BY ANTITUMOR AGENTS

The involvement of protein kinase C in transducing the elevated DAG signals of transformed cells (Fleishmann et al. 1986, Preiss et al. 1986), and of phorbol esters and other tumor promoters, renders it a candidate target for antitumor agents. The discovery or development of inhibitors of protein kinase C has the potential to further knowledge of the enzyme in growth regulation and transformation. Adriamycin (Wise et al. 1982), alkyl-lysophingolipid (Helfman et al. 1983), a nonsteroidal antiestrogen tamoxifen (O'Brian et al. 1985), and an antineoplastic lipoidal amine (Shoji et al. 1985) inhibited protein kinase C. We have discovered that the acridine class of antitumor compounds also inhibit protein kinase C (Hannun YA and Bell RM, unpublished data). The inhibition of protein kinase C by Adriamycin and by acridine orange is shown in Figure 12.5. Mechanistic studies are currently incomplete; available data suggest that acridine may inhibit by two ionic bonds between the phosphodiesters of two PS molecules present in the protein kinase C-4 PS-Ca^{2+} complex. These interactions would preclude DAG or phorbol ester from interacting to cause activation. Adriamycin may interact analogously by formation of a dimer.

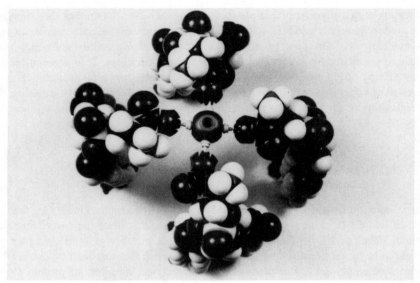

A

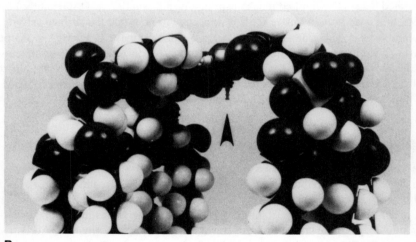

B

Figure 12.4. Model of protein kinase C activation by phospholipid, DAG, and Ca^{2+}. **A.** Overhead view of four space-filling models of PS. The four carboxyl groups are shown in close proximity to bind Ca^{2+}. Other ligands to Ca^{2+} are not shown. **B.** A view in the transverse plane of the membrane bilayer showing the complex of Ca^{2+} and four molecules of PS. An available bond to Ca^{2+} is shown unoccupied by ligand (arrow). **C.** Protein kinase C is envisioned to bind to the complex shown in **B** on the membrane surface, where it is inactive. **D.** DAG is shown to ligate directly to a Ca^{2+} present in the PS-Ca^{2+}-protein kinase C complex and, thereby, to cause activation. Activation is thought to require three points of contact, as depicted in Figure 12.3. The two remaining points could be with protein kinase C. **E.** Illustration of protein kinase C in an active state associated with a membrane as a quaternary complex with PS, DAG, and Ca^{2+}. (Figure 5 of Ganong et al. 1986b.)

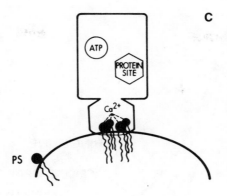

C

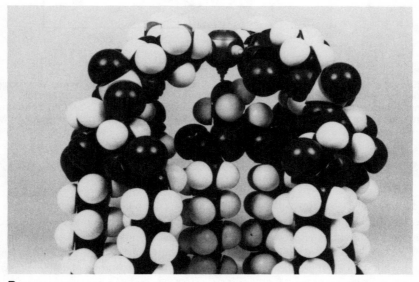

D

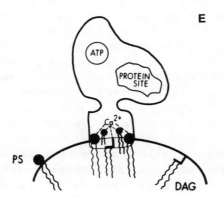

E

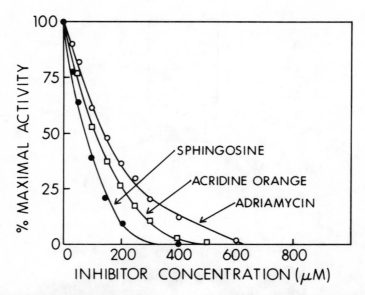

Figure 12.5. Inhibition of protein kinase C by Adriamycin, acridine orange, and sphingosine. Mixed micelles were formed with 3% (w/v) Triton X-100 containing PS at 6 mol% and $diC_{18:1}$ at 2 mol% then diluted 1:10 into the reaction mixture. Acridine orange (□) and Adriamycin (○) were added from fresh aqueous solutions. Sphingosine (●) was added with the lipid cofactors.

SPHINGOSINE INHIBITION OF PROTEIN KINASE C: POSSIBLE SECOND MESSENGER FUNCTIONS

Structure-activity studies led to the testing of ceramide as a protein kinase C effector. Although ceramide was inactive, sphingosine, a component of ceramide, proved to be about as effective an inhibitor of protein kinase C as DAG was an activator (Hannun et al. 1986b). Not only did sphingosine inhibit protein kinase C activity but it blocked phorbol ester binding in vitro and in human platelets, where it also blocked thrombin and DAG-dependent 40-kDa protein phosphorylation. The mixed micellar analyses have provided a detailed understanding of the mechanism of inhibition by sphingosine. Moreover lysosphingolipids proved to be effective inhibitors of protein kinase C; substitution at position 1 was without effect (Hannun YA and Bell RM, unpublished data). Since sphingosine/lysosphingolipids are normal cellular constituents, these observations raised the possibility that sphingosine or sphingosine derivatives may function physiologically as intracellular regulators of protein kinase C activity. The possibility that such molecules function as second messengers should be considered.

Interestingly, sphingosine inhibits the phorbol ester or DAG-dependent differentiation of HL60 cells; thus, the untested hypothesis that alteration of sphingosine levels may be the molecular basis of certain forms of human leukemia arose (Merrill et al. 1986). The activation of the oxidative burst of human neutrophils by opsonized zymosan, F-met-leu-phe, arachidonate, DAGs, and phorbol esters was inhibited by sphingosine (Wilson et al. 1986). These data establish that sphingosine inhibits protein kinase C in cells and suggest that it may be useful for investigating the function of protein kinase C in living cells in general.

These data also raise the interesting possibility that sphingosine/lysosphingolipid inhibition of protein kinase C may occur physiologically (see Fig. 12.5, Hannun et al. 1986b). Protein kinase C activity would be a function of positive (DAG) and negative (sphingosine/lysosphingolipid) levels (Hannun and Bell 1987). The presence of negative effectors of protein kinase C could explain why the enzyme is not activated by resting DAG levels. Negative effectors could alter the "set point" for protein kinase C activation in cells. The possibility that sphingosine/lysosphingolipids compose a new set of intracellular second messengers produced in response to extracellular agents should not be overlooked. These molecules could define, in part, the physiological significances of the membrane sphingolipids that have been implicated in the transformed state (Hakomori 1986).

ACKNOWLEDGMENT

This investigation was supported by grant number AM 20205 from the National Institute of Arthritis, Diabetes, Digestive, and Kidney Disease and by grant BC5-511 from the American Cancer Society.

REFERENCES

Anderson WB, Estival A, Tapiovaara H, Gopalakriskna R. 1985. Altered subcellular distribution of protein kinase C (a phorbol ester receptor). Possible role in tumor promotion and the regulation of cell growth: relationship to changes in adenylate cyclase activity. *In* Cooper DMF, Seaman KB, eds., Advances in Cyclic Nucleotide and Protein Phosphorylation Research, vol. 19. Raven Press, New York, pp. 287–306.

Berridge MJ. 1984. Inositol trisphosphate and diacylglycerol as second messengers. Biochem J 220:345–360.

Boni LT, Rando RR. 1985. The nature of protein kinase C activation by physically defined phospholipid vesicles and diacylglycerols. J Biol Chem 260:10819–10825.

Davis RJ, Ganong BR, Bell RM, Czech, MP. 1985. *sn*-1,2-Dioctanoylglycerol. A cell-permeable diacylglycerol that mimics phorbol diester action on the epidermal growth factor receptor and mitogenesis. J Biol Chem 260:1562–1566.

Delclos KB, Yeh E, Blumberg PM. 1983. Specific labeling of mouse brain membrane phospholipids with [20-³H]phorbol 12-p-azidobenzoate 13-benzoate, a photolabile phorbol ester. Proc Natl Acad Sci USA 80:3054–3058

Fleishmann LF, Chahwala SB, Cantley L. 1986. *Ras*-transformed cells: Altered levels of phosphatidylinositol-4,5-bisphosphate and catabolites. Science 231:407–410.

Ganong BR, Loomis CR, Hannun YA, Bell RM. 1986a. Regulation of protein kinase C by lipid cofactors. *In* Elson E, Frazier W, Glaser L, eds., Cell Membranes: Methods and Reviews. Plenum Publishing Corp., New York.

Ganong BR, Loomis CR, Hannun YA, Bell RM. 1986b. Specificity and mechanism of protein kinase C activation by *sn*-1,2-diacylglycerols. Proc Natl Acad Sci USA 83:1184–1188.

Hakomori SI. 1986. Glycosphingolipids. Sci Am 254(4):44–53.

Hannun YA, Loomis CR, Bell RM. 1985. Activation of protein kinase C by Triton X-100 mixed micelles containing diacylglycerol and phosphatidylserine. J Biol Chem 260:10039–10043.

Hannun YA, Bell RM. 1986. Phorbol ester binding and activation of protein kinase C on triton x-100 mixed micelles containing phosphatidylserine. J Biol Chem 261:9341–9347.

Hannun YA, Loomis CR, Bell RM. 1986a. Protein kinase C activation in mixed micelles. Mechanistic implications of phospholipid, diacylglycerol and calcium interdependencies. J Biol Chem 261:7184–7190.

Hannun YA, Loomis CR, Merrill AH, Bell RM. 1986b. Sphingosine inhibition of protein kinase C activity and of phorbol dibutyrate binding *in vitro* and in human platelets. J Biol Chem 261:12604–12609.

Hannun YA, Bell RM. 1987. Lysosphingolipid inhibition of protein kinase C: Implications in the pathogenesis of the sphingolipidoses. Science 235:670–674.

Helfman DM, Barnes KC, Kinkade JM, Volger WR, Shoji M, Kuo JF. 1983. Phospholipid-sensitive Ca^{2+}-dependent protein phosphorylation system in various types of leukemic cells from human patients and in human leukemic cell lines HL60 and K562, and its inhibition by alkyl-lysophospholipid. Cancer Res 43:2955–2961.

Kennerly DA, Parker CW, Sullivan TJ. 1979. Use of diacylglycerol kinase to quantitate picomole levels of 1,2-diacylglycerol. Anal Biochem 98:123–131.

Kishimoto A, Takai Y, Mori T, Kikkawa U, Nishizuka Y. 1980. Activation of calcium and phospholipid-dependent protein kinase by diacylglycerol, its possible relation to phosphatidylinositol turnover. J Biol Chem 255:2273–2276.

Loomis CR, Walsh JP, Bell RM. 1985. *sn*-1,2-Diacylglycerol kinase of *Escherichia coli*, purification, reconstitution and partial amino- and carboxyl-terminal analysis. J Biol Chem 260:4091–4097.

Merrill AH, Sereni A, Steven W, Hannun Y, Bell RM, Kinkade J. 1986. Inhibition of phorbol ester dependent differentiation of human promyleocytic leukemic (HL60) cells by sphinganine and other long-chain bases. J Biol Chem 261:12610–12615.

Nishizuka Y. 1983. Calcium, phospholipid turnover and transmembrane signalling. Philos Trans R Soc Lond [Biol] 302:101–112.

Nishizuka Y. 1984. The role of protein kinase C in cell surface signal transductions and tumor promotion. Nature 308:693–698.

O'Brian CA, Liskamp RM, Solomon DH, Weinstein IB. 1985. Inhibition of protein kinase C by tamoxifen. Cancer Res 45:2462–2465.

Preiss J, Loomis CR, Bishop WR, Stein R, Niedel JE, Bell RM. 1986. Quantitative measurement of *sn*-1,2-diacylglycerols present in platelets, hepatocytes and *ras*- and *sis*-transformed normal rat kidney cells. J Biol Chem 261:8597–8600.

Rozengurt E, Rodriguez-Pena A, Loombs M, Sinnett-Smith J. 1984. Diacylglycerol stimulates DNA synthesis and cell division in mouse 3T3 cells: Role of Ca^{2+}-sensitive phospholipid-dependent protein kinase. Proc Natl Acad Sci USA 81:5748–5752.

Shoji M, Vogler WR, Kuo JF. 1985. Inhibition of phospholipid/Ca^{2+}-dependent protein kinase and phosphorylation of leukemic cell proteins by CP-46,665-1, a novel antineoplastic lipoidal amine. Biochem Biophys Res Commun 127:590–595.

Walsh PJ, Bell RM. 1986. *sn*-1,2-Diacylglycerol kinase of *Escherichia coli*. Mixed micellar analysis of the phospholipid cofactor requirement and divalent cation dependence. J Biol Chem 261:6239–6247.

Wilson E, Olcott MC, Bell RM, Merrill AH, Lambeth JD. 1986. Inhibition of the oxidative burst in human neutrophils by sphingoid long-chain bases: Role of protein kinase C in activation of the burst. J Biol Chem 261:12616–12623.

Wise BC, Glass DB, Jen Chou CH, et al. 1982. Phospholipid-sensitive Ca^{2+}-dependent protein kinase from heart. J Biol Chem 257:8489–8495.

Symposium on Fundamental Cancer Research, Vol. 39.
© 1987 by the University of Texas System Cancer Center.

13. The Role of Phosphoinositides in Cell Physiology

Philip W. Majerus, Thomas M. Connolly, Theodora S. Ross,
Hidemi Ishii, and Hans Deckmyn

*Division of Hematology-Oncology, Departments of Internal Medicine and Biological
Chemistry, Washington University School of Medicine, St. Louis, Missouri 63110*

**The phosphoinositides are minor phospholipids present in all eukaryotic cells. They
are storage forms for messenger molecules that function in the transmission of signals across the cell membrane and evoke responses to extracellular agonists. The
phosphoinositides break down to liberate messenger molecules or precursors of messenger molecules. Many different compounds are formed, although the functions of
only a few are understood currently.**

Stimulation of platelets and a variety of other cells with the appropriate agonists
results in the phospholipase C–mediated cleavage of phosphatidylinositol (PI) and
the polyphosphoinositides, phosphatidylinositol-4-phosphate (PIP) and phosphatidylinositol 4,5-bisphosphate (PIP$_2$) (Majerus et al. 1984). Agonist-induced phosphoinositide metabolism generates a number of cellular messenger molecules. 1,2-
Diglyceride, the lipid product of phosphoinositide cleavage by phospholipase C,
can be further metabolized by diglyceride and monoglyceride lipase enzymes to yield
free arachidonic acid for icosanoid synthesis (Bell et al. 1979). Phosphoinositide-
derived diglyceride also serves to activate protein kinase C, a ubiquitous kinase that
phosphorylates serine and threonine residues on a variety of cellular proteins in response to agonist stimulation (Nishizuka 1984). Protein kinase C has been studied
most extensively in platelets, where phosphorylation of a 40-kDa protein follows
stimulation by physiological agonists (Lyons et al. 1975, Haslam and Lynham
1977, Sano et al. 1983). Another signal molecule generated by phosphoinositide
metabolism is inositol-1,4,5-trisphosphate (IP$_3$), one of the products of PIP$_2$ hydrolysis by phospholipase C. IP$_3$ functions as a messenger that triggers intracellular Ca^{2+}
fluxes (Berridge and Irvine 1984).

In the past year, additional water-soluble phosphoinositide metabolites have
been identified, including inositol-1,3,4,5-tetrakisphosphate and inositol-1,3,4-
trisphosphate (Batty et al. 1985, Irvine et al. 1984). These newly discovered compounds are candidates for second messengers in cells. We will review additional
phosphoinositide metabolites isolated in our laboratory and describe the enzymes
controlling synthesis and degradation of these compounds.

Dawson (1971) showed that cleavage of PI by phospholipase C produces a mixture of two water-soluble metabolites: inositol-1-phosphate (IP) and inositol-1:2-cyclic phosphate (cIP). These investigators speculated that the phosphodiester bond of the cyclic product was generated by nucleophilic attack of the 2-hydroxyl of inositol on the phosphorous atom during the phospholipase C reaction. By analogy to the PI reaction, we anticipated that cyclic 1:2 phosphate esters would be found in the phospholipase C cleavage products of PIP and PIP_2, since all three phosphoinositides are hydrolyzed by a single purified phospholipase C (Wilson et al. 1984). ^{18}O-Labeling of phosphate moieties was employed to show that cyclic phosphate esters are among the water-soluble products of polyphosphoinositide cleavage by phospholipase C (Wilson et al. 1985a). Cleavage of PIP produces inositol-1,4-bisphosphate (IP_2) and the cyclic product inositol-1:2-cyclic-bisphosphate (cIP_2), while cleavage of PIP_2 produces both IP_3 and the cyclic product inositol-1:2-cyclic-4,5-tris-phosphate (cIP_3). Under in vitro conditions, 45% of the PIP cleavage product and 36% of the PIP_2 cleavage product are cyclic. We have isolated cIP_2 and cIP_3 and established the structures of these compounds through ^{18}O-labeling of the phosphate moieties, phosphomonoesterase digestion, and fast-atom bombardment mass spectrometry (Wilson et al. 1985b). The physiologic effects of these compounds have been examined in two systems: saponin-permeabilized platelets preloaded with $^{45}Ca^{2+}$ or [^{14}C]serotonin and intact *Limulus* photoreceptor cells. We have shown that cIP_3 causes release of Ca^{2+} from permeabilized platelets but that this compound is slightly less potent than IP_3; cIP_2 does not cause Ca^{2+} release from these cells (Wilson et al. 1985b). Addition of IP_3 to permeabilized platelets results in release of [^{14}C] serotonin from granule stores (Brass and Joseph 1985). A comparison of cIP_3 to IP_3 shows that these two compounds are equipotent in ability to release [^{14}C]serotonin from labeled platelets (Fig. 13.1). Injection of cIP_3 into *Limulus* photoreceptor cells induces both a change in membrane conductance and a transient increase in intracellular Ca^{2+} similar to the conductance and increase induced by light and IP_3 (Wilson et al. 1985b). When IP_3 and cIP_3 were injected into the same photoreceptor cell, the cyclic compound was found to be approximately five times more potent than the noncyclic compound in stimulating a conductance change. No consistent change in membrane conductance was observed when cIP_2 was injected into these cells. Based on these results, we speculate that cIP_3 may function as a second messenger in stimulated cells. No specific physiological role of the cyclic compounds that is distinct from the noncyclic compounds has yet been identified.

The existence of inositol cyclic phosphate esters in intact stimulated cells has recently been documented by several investigators. cIP has been isolated from stimulated mouse pancreas cells, human platelets, and SV40 transformed mouse cells (reviewed in Ross and Majerus 1986). Recently, we isolated cIP_3 from thrombin-stimulated platelets labeled with $^{32}PO_4$ (Ishii et al. 1986). We observed cIP_3 in thrombin-treated platelets (10 sec) in each of three experiments. There was no cIP_3 formed in unstimulated platelets or in platelets incubated for 10 min with thrombin. An internal standard of [^3H]cIP_3 was used to determine the amount off [^{32}P]cIP_3 formed. The specific activity of the [^{32}P]cIP_3 was estimated by measuring the specific activity of its lipid precursor, PIP_2. Based on these measurements, we calcu-

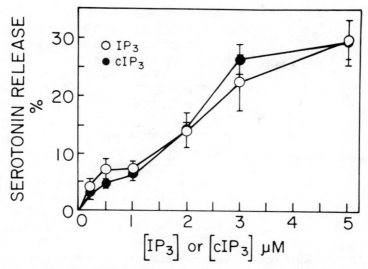

Figure 13.1. IP_3- and cIP_3-induced [^{14}C]serotonin secretion from saponin-treated platelets. Experimental procedures were the same as described elsewhere (Wilson et al. 1985b).

lated that at 10 sec after thrombin stimulation, the levels of cIP_3 were 0.22, 0.35, and 0.43 nmol/10^9 platelets in three experiments. These values are similar to the decrease in PIP_2 mass observed after thrombin stimulation and comparable to the direct measurement of IP_3 mass in stimulated platelets made by Rittenhouse and Sasson (1985) (0.17 nmol/10^9 platelets). These studies verify that inositol cyclic phosphates are produced in vivo. The relative proportion of cyclic to noncyclic product produced in cells and the relative physiological importance of these compounds is currently unknown.

Assuming that IP_3 and cIP_3 are mediators of cellular function, their degradation may be a signal-terminating step. Studies in a variety of tissues have shown that the noncyclic inositol phosphates are degraded by a series of specific phosphomono-esterases (reviewed in Connolly et al. 1986b) (Fig. 13.2). We have isolated a soluble 40-kDa phosphomonoesterase from human platelets that specifically removes the 5-phosphate moiety from IP_3 to produce IP_2 (Connolly et al. 1985). This purified phosphomonoesterase also degrades cIP_3 to produce cIP_2 (Connolly et al. 1986b). When cIP_3 is added to a crude extract of platelets, it is converted by 5-phosphomonoesterase activity into cIP_2; there is no conversion of cIP_3 into IP_3 by the cell-free extract. IP_2 and cIP_2 are degraded to IP and cIP, respectively, by the same platelet extract. In extracts of platelets and other cells IP is converted to inositol by an inositol-1-phosphatase an enzyme that is inhibited by Li^+ (Hallcher and Sherman 1980). cIP is converted to IP by inositol 1:2 cyclic phosphate-2 phosphohydrolase, an enzyme activity first described by Dawson and Clarke (1972). We have recently purified this cIP phosphohydrolase 1300-fold to homogeneity from the soluble fraction of human placenta (Ross and Majerus 1986). The enzyme re-

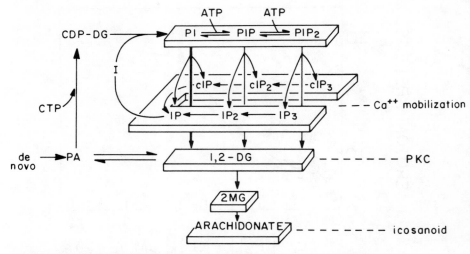

Figure 13.2. Pathways of phosphoinositide metabolism (see text for discussion).

quires Mn^{2+} or Mg^{2+} for activity, has an apparent K_m for cIP of 150 μM, and forms 2.2 μmol IP/min/mg protein. The enzyme does not use the cyclic ester of cIP_3 or cIP_2 as substrates. The molecular weight determined by gel filtration is approximately 55,000. Upon electrophoresis in sodium dodecyl sulfate (SDS) polyacrylamide gels, the molecular weight was found to be 29,000 in the presence and absence of 2-mercaptoethanol, suggesting that the protein may exist as a dimer of identical subunits. Neither Li^+ nor Ca^{2+} have any effect on enzyme activity. The existence of a specific enzyme that converts cIP to IP implies that there is an in vivo significance of the cyclic bond. The presence of an enzyme that converts the cyclic compounds to noncyclic compounds may be crucial for proper cellular function, since free inositol is needed for resynthesis of the phosphoinositides consumed during signal transduction.

Recent studies in our laboratory suggest that an additional level of regulation may control inositol phosphate degradation in stimulated platelets and other cell types. In vitro, protein kinase C phosphorylates the purified IP_3 5-phosphomonoesterase, increasing the maximal activity of the enzyme threefold without apparently altering its K_m for IP_3 (Connolly et al. 1986a). The stoichiometry of the phosphorylation was estimated to range from 0.8 to 4.3 mol [^{32}P]PO_4 per mol of IP_3 5-phosphomono-esterase in several experiments. When the IP_3 5-phosphomonoesterase was phosphorylated with [γ-^{32}P]ATP and run on SDS polyacrylamide gels, the labeled protein comigrated with the platelet 40-kDa protein phosphorylated in intact platelets in response to thrombin stimulation. Partial digestion of the labeled 5-phospho-monoesterase and 40-kDa protein labeled in intact platelets with *Staphylococcus aureus* V8 protease resulted in the formation of two major labeled peptides that were of identical size for each protein. Trypsin digestion produced three labeled peptides of identical size for each protein. From these results we conclude that the IP_3 5-phosphomonoesterase and the 40-kDa protein are the same protein. These results suggest that platelet Ca^{2+} mobilization may be regulated by protein kinase c phosphorylation of IP_3 5-phosphomonoesterase and provide a mechanism for termination of phosphoinositide-mediated signal transduction in platelets. These results also explain the observation that activation of protein kinase c in intact platelets by treatment with phorbol esters results in a decrease in the level of IP_3 and decreased Ca^{2+} mobilization upon subsequent thrombin addition.

Many questions remain to be answered concerning phosphoinositide metabolism. Future experiments may elucidate which phosphoinositide metabolites are critical to the response of cells to agonists. There is considerable interest in the role that phosphatidylinositol turnover plays in regulating cell growth. A relationship between phosphoinositides and cell growth is suggested by the finding that several growth factors, including platelet-derived growth factor and epidermal growth factor, stimulate phosphoinositide turnover (Habenicht 1981, Macara, 1986). In addition, the tumor-promoting phorbol esters stimulate protein kinase C directly, thereby bypassing the phosphoinositide-derived diacylglycerol cofactor. Thus, alterations in the phosphoinositide signal pathway could affect the control of cell growth. The stimulation of phosphoinositide turnover in the transforming process of a tumor virus was first shown in studies of Rous sarcoma virus–transformed quail cells (Diringer and Friis 1977). More recently, it was suggested that the transforming proteins of tumor viruses that are protein tyrosine kinases are also lipid kinases that could convert PI to PI 4P (Sugimoto et al. 1984, Macara et al. 1984). A difficulty with the hypothesis was that the PI kinase activity of these protein tyrosine kinases was meager compared to cellular PI kinase. Further studies have refuted the hypothesis by showing that the transforming protein tyrosine kinases are devoid of PI kinase activity (Sugano and Hanafusa 1985, Sugimoto and Erikson 1985, MacDonald et al. 1985, Fry et al. 1985). However, these studies did confirm the finding that phosphoinositide turnover is increased in transformed cells. Furthermore, membranes from v-*fms*– and v-*fes*–transformed cells have increased PI $4,5P_2$-specific phospholipase C activity compared to uninfected cells (Jackowski et al. 1986). Thus, there remains the possibility that derangements of the phosphoinositide messenger system may be important in the development of uncontrolled growth in transformed cells.

ACKNOWLEDGMENT

We thank Teresa Bross, David Wilson, and L. F. Brass who carried out some of the work described. This research was supported by grants HLBI-14147 (Specialized Center for Research in Thrombosis), HLBI-16634, and training grant T32 HLBI 07088 from the National Institutes of Health, a NATO Research Fellowship, and a Fulbright Award to Hans Deckmyn.

REFERENCES

Batty, JR, Nahorski SR, Irvine RF. 1985. Rapid formation of inositol 1,3,4,5-tetrakisphosphate following muscarinic receptor stimulation of rat cerebral cortical slices. Biochem J 232:211–215.

Bell RL, Kennerly DA, Stanford N, Majerus PW. 1979. Diglyceride lipase: A pathway for arachidonate release from human platelets. Proc Natl Acad Sci USA 76:3238–3241.

Berridge MJ, Irvine MJ. 1984. Inositol trisphosphate a novel second messenger in cellular signal transduction. Nature 312:315–321.

Brass LF, Joseph SK. 1985. A role for IP$_3$ in intracellular Ca^{2+} mobilization and granule secretion in platelets. J Biol Chem 260:15172–15179.

Connolly TM, Bross TE, Majerus PW. 1985. Isolation of a phosphomonoesterase from human platelets that specifically hydrolyzes the 5-phosphate of inositol 1,4,5-trisphosphate. J Biol Chem 260:7868–7874.

Connolly TM, Lawing WJ Jr, Majerus PW. 1986a. Protein kinase C phosphorylates human platelet inositoltrisphosphate 5'-phosphomonoesterase increasing the phosphatase activity. Cell 46:951–958.

Connolly TM, Wilson DB, Bross TE, Majerus PW. 1986b. Isolation and characterization of the inositol cyclic phosphate products of phosphoinositide cleavage by phospholipase C. II. Metabolism in cell free extracts. J Biol Chem 261:122–126.

Dawson RMC, Clarke N. 1972. D-myoinositol 1:2-cyclic phosphate 2-phosphohydrolase. Biochem J 127:113–118.

Dawson RHC, Freinkel N, Jungalwala FB, Clarke N. 1971. The enzymatic formation of inositol 1:2-cyclic from phosphatidyl inositol. Biochem J 122:605–607.

Diringer H, Friis RR. 1977. Change in phosphatidylinositol metabolism correlated to growth state of normal and RSV-transformed Japanese quail cells. Cancer Res 37:2979–2984.

Fry MJ, Gebhardt A, Parker PJ, Foulkes JG. 1985. Phosphatidylinositol turnover or transformation of cells by Abelson MLV. EMBO J 4:3173–3178.

Habenicht AJR. 1981. Early changes in phosphatidylinositol and arachidonate metabolism in quiescent 3T3 cells stimulated to divide by PDGF. J Biol Chem 256:12329–12335.

Hallcher LM, Sherman WR. 1980. The effects of *Lithium* and other agents on the activity of inositol-1-phosphatase from bovine brain. J Biol Chem 255:10896–10901.

Haslam RJ, Lynham JA. 1977. Relationship between phosphorylation of blood platelet proteins and secretion of platelet granule constituents. Biochem Biophys Res Commun 77:714–722.

Irvine RF, Letcher AJ, Lander DJ, Downes CP. 1984. Inositol trisphosphates in carbachol-stimulated rat paraotid glands. J Biochem 223:237–243.

Ishii H, Connolly TM, Bross TE, Majerus PW. 1986. Inositol cyclic trisphosphate (inositol 1:2-cyclic,4,5 trisphosphate) is formed upon thrombin stimulation of human platelets. Proc Natl Acad Sci USA 83:6397–6401.

Jackowski S, Rettenmier CW, Sherr CJ, Rock CV. 1986. A guanine nucleotide-dependent PI 4,5P$_2$ phospholipase C in cells transformed by the v-*fms* and v-*fes* oncogenes. J Biol Chem 261:4978–4985.

Lyons RM, Stanford N, Majerus PW. 1975. Thrombin-induced protein phosphorylation in human platelets. J Clin Invest 56:924–936.

Macara IG. 1986. Activation of ^{45}Ca^{2+} influx and ^{23}Na$^+$/H$^+$ exchange by EGF and vanadate in A431 cells is independent of phosphatidylinositol turnover and is inhibited by phorbol ester and diacylglycerol. J Biol Chem 261:9321–9327.

Macara IG, Marinetti GV, Balduzzi PC. 1984. Transforming protein of avian sarcoma virus UR2 is associated with phosphatidylinositol kinase activity. Proc Natl Acad Sci USA 81:2728–2732.

MacDonald ML, Keunzel EA, Glomset JA, Krebs EW. 1985. Evidence from transformed cell lines that the phosphorylations of peptide tyrosine and phosphatidylinositol are catalyzed by different proteins. Proc Natl Acad Sci USA 82:3993–3997.

Majerus PW, Neufeld EJ, Wilson DB. 1984. Production of phosphoinositide-derived messengers. Cell 37:701–703.

Nishizuka Y. 1984. The role of protein kinase C in cell surface signal transduction and tumour promotion. Nature 308:693–697.

Rittenhouse SE, Sasson JP. 1985. Mass changes in myoinositol trisphosphate in human platelets stimulated by thrombin: inhibitor effects of phorbol ester. J Biol Chem 260: 8652–8661.

Ross TS, Majerus PW. 1986. Isolation of D-*myo*-inositol 1:2 cyclic phosphate 2-inositol-phosphohydrolase from human placenta. J Biol Chem 261: 11119–11123.

Sano K, Takai Y, Yamanishi J, Nishizuka Y. 1983. A role of calcium-activated phospholipid-dependent protein kinase in human platelet activation. J Biol Chem 258: 2010–2013.

Sugano S, Hanafusa H. 1985. Phosphatidylinositol kinase activity in virus-transformed and nontransformed cells. Mol Cell Biol 5: 2399–2404.

Sugimoto Y, Erikson RL. 1985. Phosphatidylinositol kinase activities in normal and Rous sarcoma virus-transformed cells. Mol Cell Biol 5: 3194–3198.

Sugimoto Y, Whitman M, Cantley LC, Erikson RL. 1984. Evidence that the Rous sarcoma virus transforming gene product phosphorylates phosphatidylinositol and diacylglycerol. Proc Natl Acad Sci USA 81: 2117–2121.

Wilson DB, Bross TE, Hofmann SL, Majerus PW. 1984. Hydrolysis of polyphospho-inositides by purified sheep seminal vesicle phospholipase C enzymes. J Biol Chem 259: 11718–11724.

Wilson DB, Bross TE, Sherman WR, Berger RA, Majerus PW. 1985a. Inositol cyclic phosphates are produced by cleavage of polyphosphoinositides with purified sheep seminal vesicle phospholipase C enzymes. Proc Natl Acad Sci USA 82: 4013–4017.

Wilson DB, Connolly TM, Bross TE, et al. 1985b. Isolation and characterization of the inositol cyclic phosphate products of polyphosphoinositide cleavage by phospholipase C: Physiological effects in permeabilized platelets and *Limulus* photoreceptor cells. J Biol Chem 260: 13496–13501.

Symposium on Fundamental Cancer Research, Vol. 39.
© 1987 by The University of Texas System Cancer Center.

14. Phosphatidylinositol Kinases and Cell Transformation

Lewis Cantley, Malcolm Whitman, David R. Kaplan,*
Suresh B. Chahwala, Laurie Fleischman, Gerda Endemann,
Brian S. Schaffhausen,[†] and Thomas M. Roberts

*Departments of Physiology and [†]Biochemistry, Tufts University School of Medicine and
*Laboratory of Neoplastic Disease Mechanisms and Department of Pathology,
Dana-Farber Cancer Institute, Harvard Medical School, Boston, Massachusetts 02111*

Products of phosphatidylinositol (PI) turnover have recently been implicated as regulators of cell growth and differentiation. Transformation of cells in culture by infection with certain viruses (Rous sarcoma virus, Kirsten sarcoma virus, and polyoma virus) or by transfection with the oncogenes carried by these viruses affect the steady-state level of intermediates in the PI turnover pathway. In addition, immunoprecipitates of the transforming gene products of Rous sarcoma virus and polyoma virus contain activities of certain enzymes in the PI turnover pathway. We have previously reported that polyoma middle T immunoprecipitates can catalyze phosphorylation of PI to phosphatidylinositol-4-phosphate (PIP). This activity is not intrinsic to middle T or pp60$^{c\text{-src}}$ but is due to a cellular enzyme that specifically associates with the middle T/pp60$^{c\text{-src}}$ complex. The PI kinase is found in immunoprecipitates of the middle t protein from polyoma viruses that are capable of cell transformation but does not associate with mutants of middle t defective in transformation, suggesting that this association may be important for transformation. Two PI kinases from fibroblasts (type I and type II) that are separable by anion exchange chromatography have been partially purified and characterized. These enzymes differ in their K_m for ATP as well as their K_i for adenosine and ADP. Only the type I PI kinase specifically associates with the transformation-competent mutants of middle T.

A body of information has accumulated suggesting that second messengers generated from the phosphatidylinositol (PI) turnover pathway contribute to regulation of cell growth and transformation (Whitman et al. 1986). The key observation implicating this pathway was that the cellular receptor for tumor-promoting phorbol esters (agents that stimulate many of the same responses in cells as growth factors) is a calcium, phospholipid, and diacylglycerol (DAG)-activated protein kinase (C-kinase) (Castagna et al. 1982). Phorbol esters activate this enzyme by replacing the normal regulator, DAG. This observation suggested that the numerous cellular events that had been observed to occur in response to phorbol esters (including rapid changes in ion fluxes, phosphorylation of ribosomal proteins, induction of *fos* and *myc* genes, and growth-promoting activity) are mediated by this kinase. Even more interesting was the implication that elevation of cellular DAG is the critical signal for this response. The observation that several mitogens and most notably platelet-derived growth factor (PDGF) can elevate cellular DAG levels by stimulating cleavage of PI implicated the PI turnover response in growth regulation (Berridge et al. 1984).

The role of PI turnover in growth regulation became even more interesting with the discovery that it is a phosphorylated form of PI that is first broken down in response to hormones and that in addition to DAG, another second messenger is also generated, inositol 1,4,5 trisphosphate (IP_3) (Berridge and Irvine 1984). IP_3 regulates cytosolic calcium levels by stimulating calcium release from the endoplasmic reticulum. Thus, when mitogens such as PDGF bind to target cells the diacylglycerol produced from PI turnover activates C kinase and the IP_3 elevates cytosolic calcium, which in turn activates a diverse set of responses mediated by calcium-binding proteins.

Not all mitogens are capable of rapid activation of PI turnover. For example, the primary response to epidermal growth factor (EGF) appears to be calcium influx from outside the cell rather than PI turnover (Sawyer and Cohen 1981, Moolenar et al. 1986, Macara 1986), although a secondary PI turnover response occurs in some cells. In addition, it seems likely that the various growth factor receptors activate other cellular responses independent of and in parallel with the changes in PI turnover and calcium elevation (Whitman et al. 1986). What these other responses are is unclear. The mechanism by which growth factor binding to a receptor results in activation of calcium influx or PI turnover or other primary changes in the cell is still not known.

A clue to the mechanism of growth factor receptor action was provided from work on virus encoded oncogenes. In the late 1970s and early 1980s a host of transforming genes were found to encode for protein tyrosine kinases (Hunter and Cooper 1985). Phosphorylation of proteins on tyrosine is a relatively rare event and had not been previously observed. Subsequently, Cohen's group discovered that the EGF receptor has EGF-regulated tyrosine kinase activity suggesting a link between oncogenes and growth factor receptors (Cohen et al. 1982). This link became solid with the discovery that the virus encoded oncogene *erb*B is a viral homologue of the cellular EGF receptor (Downward et al. 1984). A second oncogene, *sis,* is homologous to PDGF, whose receptor is also a protein tyrosine kinase (Waterfield et al. 1983). Thus, it is now clear that many oncogenes accomplish cell transformation merely by mimicking the function of growth factors or growth-factor receptors and that activation of tyrosine kinase activity is critical for the cellular response to many growth factors and oncogenes.

The major missing piece in this puzzle has been the identification of substrates for the tyrosine kinases that are relevant to the pleiotropic responses of cells to growth factors and transforming genes. To date, the identified substrates have provided no satisfactory model. An intriguing link of tyrosine kinases to the PI turnover response was proposed when two research groups found that PI kinase activity copurified with two different oncogene-encoded tyrosine kinases, pp60[v-src] (Sugimoto et al. 1984) and pp68[v-ros] (Maraca et al. 1984). The difficulty of separating tyrosine kinase activity from PI kinase activity suggested that these may be intrinsic activities of the same protein. However, more recent results indicate that the PI kinase is a separate enzyme that specifically binds to certain activated tyrosine kinases (Kaplan et al. 1986, Whitman et al. 1987). The possibility that this PI kinase is regulated by the tyrosine kinase activity of pp60[src] is attractive since it could at least partially explain the increased flux of phosphate through intermediates of the PI turnover cycle observed in *src*- and *ros*-transformed cells (Sugimoto et al. 1984, Macara et al. 1984). The increased IP$_3$ and DAG might then explain many of the pleiotropic responses to oncogene-induced cell transformation. A model suggesting sites at which certain oncogenes may affect PI turnover and calcium influx is presented in Figure 14.1.

Our studies on polyoma virus, a DNA tumor virus, have extended previous observations on the association between transformation and both PI and PIP kinase activities and have provided genetic, biochemical and physiological evidence for a functional, rather than fortuitous, association (Kaplan et al. 1986, Whitman et al 1985). In this chapter we summarize recent evidence that fibroblasts contain two distinct PI kinases that are separable by anion exchange chromatography and that

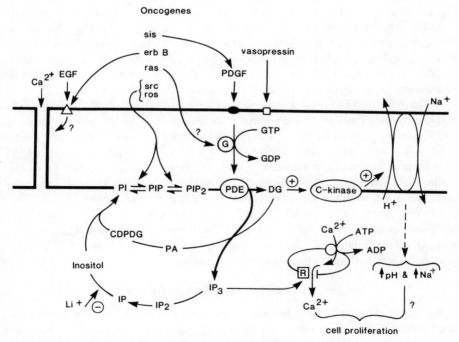

Figure 14.1. A model for potential sites of action of oncogene products on regulatory steps of phosphatidylinositol turnover and ion fluxes (see text for discussion).

have different catalytic properties. Only one of these two enzymes specifically associates with the middle T/pp60[c-src] complex.

RESULTS AND DISCUSSION

Polyoma Middle T, Tyrosine Kinase, and PI Kinase Activities

Middle T antigen is a 56–58 kDa phosphoprotein necessary for polyoma transformation (Smith and Ely 1983). A fraction of middle T associates at the inner surface of the cell membrane with pp60[c-src] (Courtneidge and Smith 1983), the cellular homologue of Rous sarcoma virus pp60[v-src]. These two proteins immunoprecipitate as a complex from polyoma-infected or transformed cells, and middle T appears to activate pp60[c-src] as a tyrosine kinase in these immunoprecipitates (Bolen et al. 1984). Transformation-defective middle T mutants fall into two categories with respect to pp60[c-src] association: those that lack normal association with pp60[c-src] and do not activate it (py1387T, NG59) and those that associate normally with pp60[c-src] at the plasma membrane and activate its tyrosine kinase activity (dl23, dl1015, 1178T, dl1014/1178T) (see Kaplan et al. 1986 for discussion).

Using immunoprecipitates made from polyoma-infected cells with an anti–polyoma T antigen antibody, we have found a phosphoinositide kinase activity associated with the middle T/pp60[c-src] complex. As shown in Table 14.1, this activity is found in immunoprecipitates made from cells infected with wild-type polyoma virus but not from cells infected with the transformation defective middle T mutant py1387T. Phosphatidylinositol 4-phosphate, but not DAG, is also phosphorylated by these immunoprecipitates (Whitman et al. 1985). Middle T/pp60[c-src]–associated PI kinase activity can also be immunoprecipitated using antibodies to c-src; in this instance, no significant PI kinase activity is associated with pp60[c-src] in the absence of transformation-competent middle T (Whitman et al. 1985).

We have assayed PI kinase activity in transformation-defective middle T mutants and have found (Table 14.1) every transformation defective mutant tested to be partially or completely defective in associated PI kinase activity. Particularly interesting are transformation defective mutants of the second category (dl23, dl1015). Immunoprecipitates of these middle T mutants phosphorylate exogenously added enolase on tyrosine at rates comparable to wild type. However, these immunoprecipitates are substantially defective in their associated PI kinase activity. The critical substrates for the middle T/pp60[c-src] tyrosine kinase in vivo are unknown, but these results indicate that for these middle T mutants transforming activity is more closely correlated with association of the complex with PI kinase activity than with tyrosine kinase activity towards an artificial substrate.

Changes in PI Metabolism in Transformed Cells

If the middle T/pp60[c-src] complex interaction with a PI kinase activity in vitro indeed reflects a regulatory interaction that is physiologically significant in vivo, expression of middle T in cells should result in an alteration in polyphosphoinositide

Table 14.1. *Transformation Mutants in the Middle T Gene of Polyoma.*
Relative Amounts of Tyrosine Kinase Activity and Phosphatidylinositol Kinase Activity
Associated with the Immunoprecipitated Middle T Protein

Polyoma Mutant	Transformation Competence	Tyrosine Kinase Activity	Increased Cell PIP	PI Kinase Activity
RA (wild-type)	+	+	+	100
Mock infected	−	−	−	7
NG59	−	−	*	10
py1387	−	−	−	8
dl23	+/−	+	*	14
dl1015	+/−	+	*	23
py1178T	+/−	+	*	23
dl1014/py1178T	+/−	+	*	19

Adapted from Kaplan et al. 1986; see Kaplan's article for details of the assays for PI kinase and tyrosine kinase.
*Not investigated.

levels in these cells. Furthermore, if polyphosphoinositide levels are important in regulating the rate of phosphoinositide turnover, levels of the inositol phosphates should also be changed upon middle T expression. We have found that both cellular polyphosphoinositide and inositol polyphosphate levels in quiescent cells are increased by expression of wild-type middle T (Table 14.1), but not by expression of the transformation defective py1387 middle T.

Although the changes in PI metabolite levels we have observed are consistent with the model for middle T action on the PI cycle that we propose, it is difficult to interpret changes in steady-state levels of intermediates as changes in the kinetics of the pathway without a full understanding of the rate-limiting steps in this pathway. Our hypothesis that middle T alters PI turnover by accelerating PI and PIP_2 phosphorylation to PIP_2, depends on the assumption that phospholipase C is not already saturated with PIP_2 in the normal cell membrane. If phospholipase is indeed saturated with PIP_2 under unstimulated conditions, accelerated PI or PI kinase activity would not result in increased IP_3 or DAG production. Although the concentration of PIP_2 in the fibroblast cell membrane can be reliably determined, the K_m of plasma membrane phospholipase C for PIP_2 at physiological concentrations of calcium is not known. Therefore the question of saturation cannot yet be answered. In resting fibroblast cells, however, the total PIP_2 per cell is approximately equal to the IP_3 per cell (Fleischman et al. 1986), indicating that the two- to threefold increase in IP_3 seen upon stimulation by serum or growth factors requires new PIP_2 synthesis. This contention is supported by a detailed kinetic analysis of GTP-γ-S–stimulated PI turnover in fibroblast cell homogenates (Chahwala et al. 1987). Direct assessment of our proposal that increased PI and PIP kinase activities caused by middle T will result in increased second messenger levels will require a more complete understanding of phospholipase C as a rate-limiting step in PI turnover. Our data do not, however, exclude the possibility that middle T directly affects phospholipase C in addition to increasing PI and PIP kinase activities.

Fibroblasts Contain Two Distinct PI Kinases

Recently we have shown that mammalian fibroblasts contain two different PI kinases, type I and type II, that are separable by anion exchange chromatography after solubilization in nonionic detergent (Whitman et al. 1987). These two enzymes have distinct kinetic properties (Table 14.2): the type II PI kinase is the more abundant of the two, is activated by addition of nonionic detergents, and is inhibited by low concentrations of adenosine and ADP. Bovine brain and human red cells also contain a PI kinase activity with properties similar to the fibroblast type II PI kinase (Endemann G, Dunn S, Cantley L, unpublished data). The type I PI kinase is less abundant in fibroblasts, is relatively insensitive to inhibition by adenosine or ADP and is reversibly inhibited by nonionic detergents. Bovine brain also contains an adenosine insensitive PI kinase that is kinetically distinguishable from either the fibroblast type I or type II PI kinases (Endemann G, Dunn S, Cantley L, unpublished data). Significantly, the polyoma middle T/pp60$^{c\text{-}src}$–associated PI kinase was identical to the type I enzyme. The PI kinase activity that specifically immunoprecipitated with pp60$^{v\text{-}src}$ was also identical to the type I enzyme (Whitman et al. 1987). Even more interesting is our observataion that this enzyme could also be precipitated from polyoma-transformed cells with antibodies directed against phosphotyrosine. These results have all suggested that the type I PI kinase or a tightly bound subunit is phosphorylated on tyrosine in polyoma-transformed cells but not in normal quiescent cells.

The amount of PI kinase activity brought down with middle T in our immunoprecipitates is only a small fraction ($\sim 1\%$) of the total PI kinase present in cell lysates (Whitman M, Kaplan DR, unpublished data). This result is partially explained by the fact that only the type I PI kinase, a minor fraction of the total activity in cell homogenates, specifically associates with this complex. However the type I PI kinase is not stoichiometrically precipitated, which leads us to speculate that the fraction of this enzyme that associates with middle t/pp60$^{v\text{-}src}$ is the enzyme that is being covalently modified (i.e., tyrosine phosphorylation) as a means of regulation. This postulate is consistent with the observation that antiphosphotyrosine antibodies precipitate the type I PI kinase. Further purification of this enzyme should allow testing of this model.

Table 14.2. *Characterization of PI Kinases in 3T3 Fibroblasts*

Property	Type I (μM)	Middle T associated (μM)	Type II (μM)
K_m (ATP)	10	12	38
K_i (adenosine)	>100	>100	16
K_i (ADP)	>100	>100	44
NP40 effect	Decrease	Decrease	Increase
Triton X100 effect	Decrease	Decrease	Increase

See Whitman et al. 1987 for details of characterization.

ACKNOWLEDGMENT

This research was supported by grants GM36133, GM36624 (L.C.), CA34722 (B.S.), and CA30002 (T.R.) from the National Institutes of Health. Lewis Cantley and Brian Schaffhausen are Established Investigators of the American Heart Association. Malcolm Whitman is a National Science Foundation predoctoral fellow and David Kaplan is a predoctoral trainee supported by NSR Award GM07196; Gerda Endemann is a Leukemia Society Fellow.

REFERENCES

Berridge M, Heslop J, Irvine JP, Brown KD. 1984. Inositoltriphosphate formation and calcium mobilization in Swiss 3T3 cells in response to platelet-derived growth factor. Biochem J 222:195–201.

Berridge MJ, Irvine RF. 1984. Inositoltris-phosphate, a novel second messenger in cellular signal transduction. Nature 312:315–321.

Bolen JB, Thiele CJ, Israel MA, Yonemoto W, Lipsich LA, Brugge JS. 1984. Enhancement of cellular *src* gene product associated tyrosyl kinase activity following polyoma virus infection and transformation. Cell 38:767–777.

Castagna M, Takai Y, Kaibuchi K, Sano K, Kikkawa V, Nishizuka Y. 1982. Direct activation of calcium activated, phospholipid-dependent protein kinase by tumor-promoting phorbol esters. J Biol Chem 257:7847–7851.

Chahwala SB, Fleischman L, Cantley L. 1987. Kinetic analysis of GTP-gamma-S effects on phosphatidylinositol turnover in NRK cell homogenates. Biochemistry 26:612–622.

Cohen S, Ushiro C, Stocsheck C, Chinkers M. 1982. A native 170,000 epidermal growth factor receptor-kinase complex from shed plasma membrane vesicles. J Biol Chem 257:1523–1528.

Courtneidge SA, Smith AE. 1983. Polyoma virus transforming protein associates with the product of the c-*src* cellular gene. Nature 303:435–439.

Downward J, Yarden Y, Mayes E, et al. 1984. Close similarity of epidermal growth factor receptor and v-erb-B oncogene product sequences. Nature 307:521–527.

Fleischman LF, Chahwala SB, Cantley L. 1986. *Ras*-transformed cells: Altered levels of phosphatidylinositol-4,5-bisphosphate and catabolites. Science 231:407–410.

Hunter T, Cooper J. 1985. Protein-tyrosine kinases. Annu Rev Biochem 54:897–930.

Kaplan DK, Whitman MR, Schaffhausen B, et al. 1986. Polyphosphoinositide metabolism and polyoma mediated transformation. Proc Natl Acad Sci USA 83:3624–3628.

Macara IG. 1986. Activation of $^{45}Ca^{2+}$ influx and $^{22}Na^+/H^+$ exchange by epidermal growth factor and vanedate in A431 cells is independent of phosphatidylinositol turnover and is inhibited by phorbol ester and diacylglycerol. J Biol Chem 261:9321–9327.

Macara, IG, Marinetti GV, Balduzzi PC. 1984. Transforming protein of avian sarcoma virus UR2 is associated with phosphatidylinositol kinase activity: Possible role in tumorigenesis. Proc Natl Acad Sci USA 81:2728–2732.

Moolenar WH, Aerts RJ, Tertoolen LGJ, de Laat SW. 1986. The epidermal growth factor induced calcium signal in A-431 cells. J Biol Chem 261:279–284.

Sawyer ST, Cohen S. 1981. Enhancement of calcium uptake and phosphatidylinositol turnover by epidermal growth factor in A-431 cells. Biochem 20:6280–6286.

Smith AE, Ely BK. 1983. The biochemical basis of transformation by polyoma virus. *In* Klein G, ed., Advances in Viral Oncology, vol. 3. New York, Raven Press, pp. 3–30.

Sugimoto Y, Whitman M, Cantley LC, Erikson RL. 1984. Evidence that the Rous sarcoma transforming gene product phosphorylates phosphatidylinositol and diacylglycerol. Proc Natl Acad Sci USA 81:2117–2121.

Waterfield MD, Scrace GT, Whittle N. et al. 1983. Platelet derived growth factor is structurally related to the putative transforming protein p28 *sis* of simian sarcoma virus. Nature 304:35–38.

Whitman M, Fleischman L, Chahwala S, Cantley L, Rosoff P. 1986. Phosphoinositides, mitogenesis and oncogenesis. *In* Putney JW, ed., Phosphoinositides and Receptor Mechanisms. New York, Alan R. Liss, Inc., pp. 197–217.

Whitman M, Kaplan D, Roberts T, Cantley L. 1987. Evidence for two distinct Phosphatidylinositol kinases in fibroblasts: Implications for cellular regulation. Biochem J (in press).

Whitman M, Kaplan DR, Schaffhausen B, Cantley L, Roberts TM. 1985. Association of phosphatidylinositol kinase activity with polyoma middle-T competent for transformation. Nature 315:239–242.

Symposium on Fundamental Cancer Research, Vol. 39.
© 1987 by The University of Texas System Cancer Center.

15. Studies on the Mechanism of Action of Protein Kinase C and the Isolation of Molecular Clones Encoding the Enzyme

I. Bernard Weinstein, Catherine A. O'Brian, Gerard M. Housey,
Mark D. Johnson, Paul Kirschmeier, and Wendy Hsiao

*Comprehensive Cancer Center and Institute of Cancer Research,
Columbia University College of Physicians and Surgeons,
New York, New York 10032*

Protein kinase C (PKC) plays an important role in signal transduction and the action of phorbol ester tumor promoters, and it is of interest to isolate the coding sequence of this enzyme. Using a 53-base pair synthetic oligonucleotide probe that corresponds to an 18-amino acid peptide obtained from rat brain PKC, we have isolated rat brain cDNA clones corresponding to PKC. We have also isolated several closely related clones. Partial nucleotide sequence analysis of one of the PKC clones (RP41) identifies a 224-amino acid region with approximately 40% homology to the carboxy terminal and catalytic domains of both the cAMP-dependent and cGMP-dependent protein kinases. The levels of mRNA homologous to RP41 are very high in brain; very low but detectable levels are present in heart and liver. A second cDNA (RP16) was only partially sequenced, and based on its predicted amino acid sequence, it shares 65% homology with the corresponding region of the PKC clone RP41. The levels of mRNA corresponding to RP16 are also highest in rat brain, but they are of a different size than those detected with RP41. These and additional results indicate that the gene for the enzyme PKC shares considerable homology with other protein kinases and that PKC itself may belong to a new multigene family. The availability of these cDNA clones should greatly facilitate further studies on the role of PKC in growth control, differentiation, and multistage carcinogenesis.

Because of the central role of protein kinase C (PKC) in signal transduction, growth control, and tumor promotion (for review, see Nishizuka 1986, O'Brian et al. 1986a, Weinstein 1987) researchers in our laboratory have extensively studied the function of PKC and have also cloned DNA sequences that encode this enzyme. Figure 15.1 presents a hypothetical diagram of PKC, emphasizing the fact that the enzyme has two domains, a catalytic domain containing an ATP-binding site and the region to which protein substrates bind and a regulatory domain which is controlled by allosteric cofactors (i.e. lipid, Ca^{2+} and diacylglycerol [DAG] or lipid and 12-0-

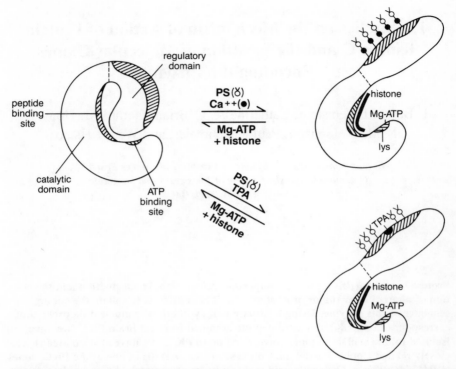

Figure 15.1. A hypothetical model of protein kinase C (PKC) emphasizing a catalytic domain that contains the ATP and peptide substrate binding sites and a regulatory domain that binds phosphatidylserine (PS) (or other lipids) and Ca²⁺, or PS and TPA. We postulate that binding of PS and Ca²⁺, or PS plus TPA, to the regulatory domain induces a conformational change in the enzyme that "opens" the catalytic domain, thus activating the phosphorylation of a protein substrate, for example histone H1. (Reprinted from Weinstein 1986, with permission.)

tetradecanoylphorbol-13-acetate [TPA]). We hypothesized that the usual function of the regulatory domain is to inactivate the enzyme by "closing" the catalytic site and that the binding of cofactors to the regulatory domain induces a conformational change that opens the catalytic site and thus activates enzyme function. Consistent with this scheme is evidence that limited proteolysis of the enzyme yields a fragment of about 66 kDa that is active in the absence of lipid and other allosteric cofactors (Girard et al. 1986). In addition, there exist inhibitors of PKC that appear to act preferentially on the regulatory domain or the catalytic domain of the enzyme (O'Brian et al. 1986a). The development of pharmacologic agents that specifically inhibit PKC could provide a novel and nonmutagenic strategy of cancer therapy. For this reason, we have also been actively engaged in developing specific inhibitors of this enzyme. We shall discuss this aspect of our work at the end of this chapter.

MOLECULAR CLONING OF DNA SEQUENCES ENCODING PROTEIN KINASE C

The Design of an Oligonucleotide Probe for cDNA's Encoding PKC

Molecular studies of PKC would be tremendously enhanced by having available cloned genes for this enzyme. We have, therefore, isolated a series of cDNA clones corresponding to PKC (Housey et al. 1986, 1987, Weinstein 1987). The general strategy that we used was as follows. PKC was partially purified from rat brain to a specific activity of 120 nmol ^{32}P/min/mg. The enzyme was then labeled with phosphorus-32 by stimulating its autophosphorylation activity and subjected to preparative polyacrylamide gel electrophoresis and autoradiography, and the ^{32}P-labeled enzyme was identified as a homogeneous 82-kDa band. This band was then excised from the gel and the protein was recovered by electroelution. The purified enzyme was reduced, carboxymethylated, dialyzed, and cleaved with endoproteinase Lys C. Cleavage peptides were separated by reverse-phase high pressure liquid chromatography (HPLC). The sequence of one of these peptides, K-S-V-D-W-W-A-F-G-V-L-L-Y-E-M-L-A-G-Q (peptide P2), was used to design an oligonucleotide probe.

Isolation of cDNA Clones Homologous to a PKC Probe

Initial screening of 6×10^5 clones from a rat brain gt10 cDNA library identified 41 clones that hybridized under low-stringency conditions to the above described ^{32}P-labeled oligonucleotide probe. These clones were isolated and placed into distinct groups based upon the intensity of their hybridization signal, restriction mapping, and high-stringency Southern blot analyses of rat genomic DNA. Thus far, we have identified five distinct groups of cDNA clones and are in the process of sequencing representatives of each group and analyzing their expression levels in various tissues. Detailed studies on two of these clones, a group I cDNA designated RP41 and a group II cDNA designated RP16, are described below.

Sequence Analysis of the cDNA Clone RP41

Restriction enzyme mapping of the RP41 clone indicated that it contains a 1.7-kb cDNA insert. Restriction fragments were subcloned into M13 vectors, and the complete nucleotide sequence of RP41 was determined. The sequence of the 720 base pair *Pst*I fragment of RP41 is shown in Figure 15.2. This sequence displays a 224 amino acid open reading frame followed by a stop codon (TAG) and includes a region of 19 amino acids that is identical with the PKC peptide P2. The latter finding, coupled with findings described below, provide strong evidence that the RP41 clone encodes the carboxy terminal region and catalytic domain of rat brain PKC. It is of particular interest that this sequence also exhibits homology with several domains present in almost all of the previously characterized protein kinases (Hunter and Cooper 1985), including the conserved amino acid clusters RDL, DFG, CGT, and APE (amino acids 18-20, 37-39, 55-57, and 62-64 in Fig. 15.2). Computer searches of the Protein Information Resource (PIR) data base, using the coding region of RP41 shown in Figure 15.2, indicated that the greatest homologies in amino

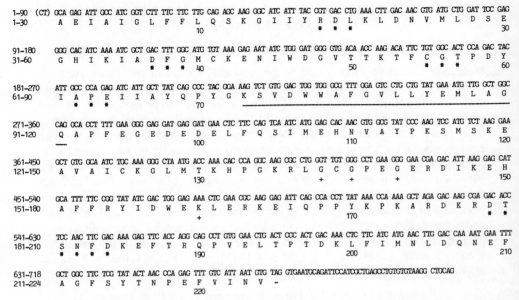

Figure 15.2. Nucleotide and deduced amino acid sequences of the cDNA clone RP41. A 720 base pair Pst I fragment encoding the 224–amino acid carboxy terminal region of rat brain PKC is displayed. Asterisks denote amino acid residues conserved among previously described protein kinases. The 19–amino acid sequence that is underlined corresponds exactly to PKC peptide P2. Amino acids that appear to constitute an ATP binding site consensus sequence are denoted with a plus (+) sign (aa 138, 140, 143, and 160).

acid sequence (about 40% overall identity) were with the catalytic subunit of the cyclic AMP-dependent protein kinase (PKA) and the carboxy terminal (catalytic) domain of the cyclic GMP–dependent protein kinase (PKG). These sequence homologies provide strong evidence that the carboxy terminal region of RP41 constitutes the catalytic domain of PKC.

Sequence Analysis of the cDNA Clone RP16

Restriction enzyme mapping of a second cDNA clone, RP16, indicated that it contains a 2.0-kb cDNA insert. Appropriate restriction fragments were subcloned into M13 vectors, and the complete nucleotide sequence of RP16 was determined. Figure 15.3 shows a 720-nucleotide segment of this sequence, along with the deduced amino acid sequence, beginning 18 amino acids upstream from an ATP-binding site consensus sequence; GXGXXG-(16 amino acids)-K (amino acids 19-21 and 41 in Fig. 15.3). As with RP41, RP16 also exhibits all of the homology domains that have been previously identified in other protein kinases, including the RDL, DFG, CGT, and APE clusters (amino acids 135-137, 154-156, 172-174, and 179-181, respectively, in Fig. 15.3). Furthermore, in the region corresponding to the PKC peptide P2 (amino acids 190-208 in Fig. 15.3) this clone differs from RP41 at only four

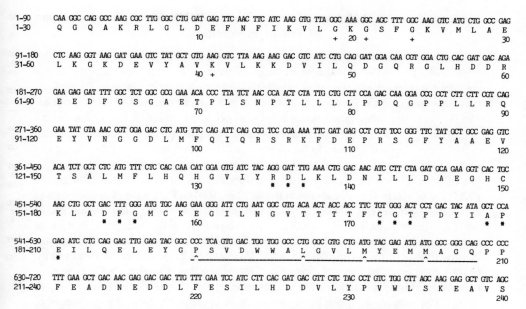

Figure 15.3. Nucleotide and deduced amino acid sequence of cDNA clone RP16. A partial sequence of RP16, a PKC-related cDNA clone, is displayed. Notations are as described in the legend to Figure 15.2. The 19–amino acid sequence underlined (aa 190-208) is identical to PKC peptide P2 at 15 of 19 positions. Arrowheads denote the four amino acids that differ between P2 and the corresponding region of RP16.

positions. The sequence of RP16 in Figure 15.3 displays 65% identity with the carboxy terminal region of RP41, whereas the homology between this region of RP41 and either PKA or PKG is only about 40%.

Analysis of the Transcripts Related to RP41 and RP16

Utilizing a ^{32}P-labeled probe prepared from the coding region of the PKC cDNA clone RP41 for northern blot analyses, we detected very high levels of two distinct transcripts of about 9 kb and 3.5 kb in the poly(A)[+] RNA fraction of rat brain. When the same poly(A)[+] RNA samples were hybridized to a ^{32}P-labeled probe prepared from the PKC-related cDNA clone RP16, a single transcript that was approximately 7.5 kb in size was detected (data not shown). The abundance of the transcripts for both RP41 and RP16 were high in brain, with moderate levels in heart and liver (Housey et al. 1987). The relative abundance of the RP41 transcript in these three tissues is consistent with published data on the levels of PKC enzymatic activities and also with the amounts of PKC protein detected in these tissues by immunoassay (Girard et al. 1986, Minakuchi et al. 1981). It will be of interest to determine whether or not there is differential expression of the individual PKC genes in various tissues and tumors.

Evidence for a PKC Multigene Family and Its Relevance to the Mechanism of Tumor Promotion

We have observed much greater homology between the PKC cDNA clone RP41 and the cDNA clone RP16 than between either of these DNA sequences and the corresponding sequences of other structurally characterized protein kinases. These findings provide evidence for the existence of a PKC multigene family (Housey et al. 1987). Recently, other laboratories have also obtained evidence for a PKC multigene family. Ono et al. (1986) have isolated and partially sequenced a rat brain cDNA clone, which appears to be identical to our clone RP41, and they have obtained peptide sequence data that suggest the existence of other forms of PKC. Knopf et al. (1986) have also partially characterized a rat brain cDNA (designated PKC III), which is virtually identical to our clone RP41. They have also isolated and completely sequenced cDNAs encoding two other forms of PKC, designated PKC I and PKC II. We have recently analyzed the 5′ terminus of a full-length cDNA clone corresponding to our clone RP41 (unpublished studies) and find that its 5′ terminus is very similar to the 5′ terminus of PKC II described by Knopf et al. Parker et al. (1986) have reported the isolation of a cDNA encoding a bovine PKC, as well as two other closely related bovine and human cDNA sequences (Coussens et al. 1986). The sequences of the latter clones differ appreciably from the sequences of our RP41 and RP16 clones. Thus, there is now substantial evidence for the existence of a PKC-related multigene family that in the rat may contain four and possibly more types of genes.

As discussed above, the present studies with PKC, and previous studies with other serine and threonine kinases and also with tyrosine protein kinases, reveal striking homologies among these protein kinases. Presumably these homologies represent their evolution from a common ancestral form. Thus, in several the catalytic domain is located in the carboxy terminal end of the molecule, whereas the regulatory domain is at the amino terminal end or is a separate protein subunit. It appears, therefore, that during evolution the amino terminal end of these proteins has undergone considerable divergence (in the case of PKA it is a separate polypeptide chain; in the case of the epidermal growth factor [EGF] receptor, it contains an extracellular EGF-binding region), thus providing regulation of the different protein kinases by quite diverse agonists. Depending on the particular kinase, the regulatory domain is responsive to the following agonists: cAMP in the case of PKA, cGMP in the case of PKG, Ca^{2+} in the case of the myosin light-chain kinase (which is regulated by calmodulin), and EGF in the case of the EGF receptor. We plan studies to determine whether deletion of the regulatory domain of PKC by recombinant DNA methods will, following transfection into mammalian cells, produce a protein that is autonomous and, therefore, cause disturbances in growth control. These studies will test the possibility that PKC can function as a proto-oncogene during carcinogenesis.

The existence of a PKC-related gene family may have several important implications with respect to growth control and tumor promotion. The existence of multiple forms of PKC may account for previously described discrepancies between the potencies of certain compounds in the activation of PKC in vitro and in tumor promotion in vivo, since various forms of PKC may have preferential sensitivity to different tumor promoters. There is precedence for a division of labor within a protein kinase family. The cAMP-dependent protein kinases fall into two major classes, type I and type II, which differ in their mechanisms of regulation and their tissue distribution (Flockhart and Corbin 1982). It seems likely that future studies employing the recently isolated PKC cDNA clones will clarify the role of this new multigene family in signal transduction, growth control, and tumor promotion. The availability of these cDNA clones may also facilitate studies concerned with the possible role of PKC in the mechanism of action of other classes of tumor promoters, for example the role of bile acids in colon carcinogenesis (Fitzer et al. 1987).

NUCLEAR EVENTS RESULTING FROM THE ACTIVATION OF PKC

A major gap in our knowledge of pathways of signal transduction is the question of how signals are conveyed from the cytoplasm to the nucleus. In the case of PKC it seems unlikely that the enzyme itself is translocated to the nucleus because attempts to demonstrate significant levels of the enzyme in the nucleus, using either TPA tagged with a fluorescent dansyl residue (Liskamp et al. 1985) or immunofluorescence with PKC antibody (Nishizuka 1986), have been negative. Another unsolved problem is the question of how, during the process of tumor promotion, the imprint of a tumor promoter becomes fixed so that the cells eventually remain abnormal even when the tumor promoter is no longer applied. If the only function of TPA is to activate PKC, then one would expect cells to revert to their previous state when the cells are no longer exposed to the tumor promoter.

We have found that when mouse or rat fibroblast cell lines are transfected with an activated H-*ras* oncogene and grown in the presence of TPA, the tumor promoter markedly enhances the yield of transformed foci (Hsiao et al. 1984, 1986). This finding has been confirmed and extended to early-passage rodent cells (Dotto et al. 1985). Since the cells obtained from these foci remain transformed, even in the absence of TPA, this system may be useful for analyzing mechanisms underlying the stable effects of TPA on cells. TPA can also enhance the transformation of adenovirus-infected rat embryo fibroblasts (Fisher et al. 1979), and it induces anchorage-independent growth of the JB6 mouse keratinocyte cell line (Colburn et al. 1979). Both of these effects are also irreversible, but the underlying mechanisms are not known.

One approach to understanding the mechanisms by which tumor promoters alter nuclear functions and gene expression is to identify the specific DNA sequences whose expression is modulated by TPA. We have, therefore, recently carried out a series of studies in which we isolated DNA sequences whose transcription is modulated in cells undergoing a mitogenic response to TPA, by differential screening of a cDNA library derived from TPA-treated cells (Johnson et al. 1986, 1987). Thus far, we have isolated and characterized two cDNA clones designated TPA-S1 and TPA-R1. TPA-S1 corresponds to an mRNA species whose abundance is markedly increased in quiescent C3H 10T1/2 mouse embryo fibroblasts exposed to TPA, whereas TPA-R1 corresponds to an mRNA species whose abundance is markedly decreased in TPA-treated cells. Thus, treatment of cells with TPA results in increased expression of certain genes and decreased expression of others. We believe that this reflects the operation of both positive and negative factors in the process of growth control (Weinstein 1987).

Detailed studies with TPA-S1 indicate that there is a marked increase in the corresponding mRNA within 1 hr after TPA treatment. The induction is blocked by actinomycin D and is specific for phorbol esters with tumor-promoting activity. The transcription of this sequence is not induced by cycloheximide (Johnson et al. 1987), as is the case for c-*myc*, c-*fos*, *actin* and certain other mitogen-induced genes (Greenberg et al. 1986). The role of PKC in the induction of TPA-S1 is supported by the following line of evidence: (1) agents that activate PKC, such as TPA, mezerein, platelet-derived growth factor (PDGF), serum, and 1-oleoyl-2-acetylglycerol (OAG), also increase TPA-S1 mRNA levels, (2) the compound H7, an inhibitor of PKC, blocks the ability of TPA to induce TPA-S1 transcripts, and (3) down-regulation of PKC activity by pretreatment of cells with TPA for 24 hr results in a loss of the ability of TPA subsequently to induce an increase in TPA-S1 transcripts. The complete sequence analysis of TPA-S1 (730 bp) predicts a cysteine-rich secreted protein with a molecular weight of 22.6 kDa. The sequence of TPA-S1 exhibits homology with sequences representing a peptide with human erythroid-potentiating activity, a human metalloproteinase inhibitor protein and a murine protein with β-interferon-like activity. Further analysis of the mechanisms underlying regulation of the TPA-S1 and TPA-R1 genes may contribute to a general understanding of how TPA treatment of cells, and the activation of PKC, alters gene expression and growth control.

INHIBITORS OF PKC

We have studied PKC inhibitors with three major objectives: (1) to acquire a more refined understanding of the mechanism of regulation of PKC, (2) to develop specific PKC inhibitors that could allow a specific pharmacologic manipulation of PKC in intact cells, and (3) to develop antiproliferative drugs. The mechanism of regulation of PKC activity is quite complex, since the phosphotransferase reaction involves two substrates (ATP and a target protein) and several cofactors (phospholipid, Ca^{2+}, TPA, diacylglycerol, Mg^{2+}), and yet the enzyme is a single polypeptide chain. Our hypothetical scheme for the activation of PKC (Fig. 15.1) predicts the possibility of developing two different classes of inhibitors of the enzyme. One class of inhibitors would act on the regulatory domain and might maintain the enzyme in the closed or "off" state, whereas, another class of inhibitors would act at the catalytic domain and interfere directly with the phosphotransferase reaction. We have found that the antiestrogen tamoxifen (and certain structurally related triphenylethylenes) and the compound rhodamine 6G are inhibitors of PKC, and we have obtained evidence that they do so by acting at the regulatory domain (O'Brian et al. 1985, 1986a,b, 1987). Tamoxifen is of interest because it is useful in the treatment of breast cancer. Although it is known to compete with estrogens for binding to the estrogen receptor, there is reason to believe that its cytotoxic effects might be due to action at sites other than the estrogen receptor (O'Brian et al. 1985). The compound rhodamine 6G is of interest because it is selectively toxic to carcinoma cells in vitro (Lampidis et al. 1985). In studies with rhodamine 6G we have found that the inhibition of PKC is markedly affected by the structure of the lipid cofactor. For example, inhibition by rhodamine 6G was 10-fold greater when the lipid cofactor was arachidonic acid rather than phosphatidylserine (O'Brian et al. 1987). Thus, the lipid microenvironment within various cell types could profoundly affect the ability of certain drugs to inhibit PKC in vivo. Tamoxifen and structurally related triphenylethylenes and rhodamine 6G have in common the property that they are amphiphilic cations. In this sense they are similar to several other amphiphilic compounds that also inhibit PKC (Mori et al. 1980, Donnelly et al. 1983). We should stress that these amphiphilic compounds are not absolutely specific as inhibitors of PKC, since some of them also inhibit other enzymes, for example calmodulin-dependent enzyme systems. These compounds may represent, however, useful prototypes for the design of more specific inhibitors of PKC.

We have also previously described studies on defined polypeptides as substrates and inhibitors of PKC (O'Brian et al. 1984). This approach could lead to the development of specific inhibitors that act at the catalytic domain of PKC. The homology between the catalytic domains of PKC, PKA, and PKG (see the discussion above) suggests that it may be difficult to obtain an inhibitor that acts at the catalytic domain but has absolute specificity for PKC. Nevertheless, this approach is worthy of pursuit.

As stressed earlier in this chapter, the development of specific inhibitors of PKC could provide a powerful new approach to the control of cell proliferation. In view of the ubiquitous role of PKC in other physiologic processes, PKC inhibitors might also have broader applications in therapeutics. The availability of molecular clones of the multiple forms of PKC should facilitate the development of such inhibitors.

ACKNOWLEDGMENT

We acknowledge the excellent secretarial assistance of Mrs. Nancy Mojica and Ms. Lintonia Sheppard. These studies were supported by NIH grant CA 02656 and funds from the Alma Toorock Memorial for Cancer Research. G. M. Housey is supported by the Medical Scientist Training Program. We thank Janusz Wideman, Stan Stein, and May Chang for valuable assistance in obtaining the amino acid data on PKC, and Cheryl Fitzer and James Murphy for valuable technical assistance.

REFERENCES

Colburn NH, Former BF, Nelson KA, Yuspa SH. 1979. Tumor promoter induces anchorage independence irreversibly. Nature 281:589–591.
Coussens L, Parker PJ, Rhee L, et al. 1986. Multiple, distinct forms of bovine and human protein kinase C suggest diversity in cellular signaling pathways. Science 233:859–866.

Donnelly TE, Jensen R. 1983. Effect of Fluphenazine on the stimulation of calcium-sensitive, phospholipid-dependent protein kinase by TPA. Life Sci 33:2247–2253.

Dotto GP, Parada LF, Weinberg RA. 1985. Specific growth response of *ras*-transformed embryo fibroblasts to tumor promoter. Nature 318:472–475.

Fisher PB, Bozzone JH, Weinstein IB 1979. Tumor promoters and epidermal growth factor stimulate anchorage-independent growth of adenovirus transformed rat embryo cells. Cell 18:695–705.

Fitzer CJ, O'Brian CA, Guillem JG, Weinstein IB. 1987. The regulation of protein kinase C by chenodeoxycholate, deoxycholate and several related bile acids. Carcinogenesis 8: 217–220.

Flockhart DA, Corbin JD. 1982. Regulatory mechanisms in the control of protein kinases. CRC Crit Rev Biochem 12:133–186.

Girard PR, Mazzei GJ, Kuo JF. 1986. Immunological quantitation phospholipid/Ca^{2+}-dependent protein kinase and its fragments. J Biol Chem 261:370–375.

Greenberg ME, Hermanowski AL, Ziff EB. 1986. Effect of protein synthesis inhibitors in growth factor activation of c-fos, c-myc and actin gene transcription. Mol Cell Biol 6: 1050–1057.

Housey GM, O'Brian CA, Johnson MD, Kirschmeier PT, Roth JS, Weinstein IB. 1986. Isolation and nucleotide sequence analysis of cDNA clones from rat brain using oligonucleotide probes to protein kinase C and protein kinase A (Abstract). J Cell Biochem 10C(Suppl):132.

Housey GM, O'Brian CA, Johnson MD, Kirschmeier PT, Weinstein IB. 1987. Isolation of cDNA clones encoding protein kinase C: Evidence for a novel protein kinase C-related gene family. Proc Natl Acad Sci USA 84:1065–1069.

Hsiao W-LW, Gattoni-Celli S, Weinstein IB. 1984. Oncogene-induced transformation of C3H 10T1/2 cells is enhanced by tumor promoters. Science 226:552–555.

Hsiao W-LW, Wu T, Weinstein IB. 1986. Oncogene-induced transformation of a rat embryo fibroblast cell line is enhanced by tumor promoters. Mol Cell Biol 6:1943–1950.

Hunter T, Cooper A. 1985. Protein-tyrosine kinases. Annu Rev Biochem 54:897–930.

Johnson MD, Housey GM, Kirschmeier P, Weinstein IB. 1986. Isolation of DNA sequences whose transcription is induced by TPA (Abstract). J Cell Biochem 10C(Suppl):133.

Johnson MD, Housey GM, Kirschmeier P, Weinstein IB. 1987. Molecular cloning of gene sequences regulated by tumor promoters and mitogens through protein kinase C. Mol Cell Biol (in press).

Knopf JL, Lee M-H, Sultzman LA, et al. 1986. Cloning and expression of multiple protein kinase C cDNAs. Cell 46:491–502.

Lampidis TJ, Hasin Y, Weiss MJ, Chen LB. 1985. Selective killing of carcinoma cells *in vitro* by lipophilic cationic compounds: A cellular basis. Biomed Pharmacother 39: 220–226.

Liskamp RMJ, Brothman AR, Arcoleo JP, Miller OJ, Weinstein IB. 1985. Cellular uptake and localization of fluorescent derivatives of phorbol ester tumor promoters. Biochem Biophys Res Commun 131:920–927.

Minakuchi R, Takai Y, Yu B, Nishizuka Y. 1981. Widespread occurrence of calcium-activated, phospholipid-dependent protein kinase in mammalian tissue. J Biochem 89: 1651–1654.

Mori T, Takai Y. Minakuchi R, Yu B, Nishizuka Y. 1980. Inhibitory action of chlorpromazine, dibucaine and other phospholipid-interacting drugs on calcium-activated, phospholipid-dependent protein kinase. J Biol Chem 255:8378–8380.

Nishizuka Y. 1986. Perspectives on the roles of protein kinase C in stimulus-response coupling. JNCI 76:363–370.

O'Brian CA, Lawrence DS, Kaiser ET, Weinstein IB. 1984. Protein kinase C phosphorylates the synthetic peptide Arg-Arg-Lys-Ala-Ser-Gly-Pro-Pro-Val in the presence of phospholipid plus either Ca^{2+} or a phorbol ester tumor promoter. Biochem Biophys Res Commun 124:296–302.

O'Brian CA, Liskamp RM, Solomon DH, Weinstein IB. 1985. Inhibition of protein kinase C by tamoxifen. Cancer Res 45:2462–2465.

O'Brian CA, Liskamp RM, Arcoleo JP, Hsiao W-LW, Housey GM, Weinstein IB. 1986a. Current concepts of tumor promoters by phorbol esters and related compounds. *In* Poste G, Crooke ST, eds., New Insights into Cell and Membrane Transport Processes. Plenum Publishing Co., New York, pp. 261–274.

O'Brian CA, Liskamp RM, Solomon DH, Weinstein IB. 1986b. Triphenylethylenes: A new class of protein kinase C inhibitors. JNCI 76:1243–1246.

O'Brian CA, Weinstein IB. 1987. The inhibition of protein kinase C, whether under the regulation of phosphatidylserine or of arachidonic acid, by Rhodamine 6G. Biochem Pharmacol (in press).

Ono Y, Kurodawa T, Kawahara K, et al. 1986. Cloning of rat brain protein kinase C complementary cDNA. FEBS Lett 203:111–115.

Parker PJ, Coussens L, Totty N, et al. 1986. The complete primary structure of protein kinase C—the major phorbol ester receptor. Science 233:853–859.

Weinstein IB. 1987. Growth factors, oncogenes and multistage carcinogenesis. J Cell Biochem 33:213–224.

SYMPOSIUM SUMMARY

Symposium on Fundamental Cancer Research, Vol. 39.
© 1987 by The University of Texas System Cancer Center.

16. The Molecular Determinants of Carcinogenesis: A Symposium Sketch

Henry C. Pitot

McArdle Laboratory for Cancer Research, Departments of Oncology and Pathology, The Medical School, University of Wisconsin, Madison, Wisconsin 53706

This monograph has emphasized the molecular aspects of both the differences between cancer and normal cells and the development of a cancer cell from a normal cell. Multistage carcinogenesis is now well known in a variety of histogenetic circumstances, and definable stages of initiation, promotion, and progression have been identified. Activation of proto-oncogenes in neoplasms may occur at any time during the development of malignancy, but most examples to date have shown this occurrence during the final stage of progression. A new form of carcinogenesis, that induced by specific genetic constructions in vivo or in vitro, has now been accomplished. The specificity of genetic carcinogenesis can reside in the specific construct itself, especially in tissue-specific enhancer regions. On the other hand, the specific molecular genetic characteristics of at least one human genetic condition resulting in a high incidence of a specific histogenetic type of neoplasia, hereditary neuroblastoma, have been partially characterized. All of the various types of carcinogenesis—genetic, viral, chemical, and radiation—exhibit, at one time or another or in one situation or another, multiple stages in their development.

Although it is possible to treat cancer with varying degrees of success, we still do not understand all of the molecular events leading up to and uniquely distinguishing the cancer cell—*any* cancer cell—from its normal counterpart. This statement, while undoubtedly correct, is not an occasion for despair but rather a framework around which future studies may develop. This framework consists of two questions at the heart of understanding the malignant process in living cells. These are:

1. How does a cancer cell differ from its normal cell of origin?
2. How does a cancer cell develop from a normal cell?

The answers to the first question are the motivation for the study of molecular oncology, an understanding of the cancer cell in molecular terms as it differs from its normal cell of origin. The answers to the second question may be derived from the field of molecular carcinogenesis, the topic of this symposium. In some instances the answers to these two questions may be similar, if not identical. Such is the case with certain cancers that are induced rapidly by small RNA viruses or DNA viruses, or both. A prime example is the infection of chickens by the Rous sarcoma virus, resulting in the rapid, disseminated development of sarcomas and death of the birds within two or three weeks (Beard 1980). Similarly, infection of young mammals by other RNA or DNA oncogenic viruses may induce disseminated malignant and fatal neoplasia within a matter of days or weeks. In view of our knowledge of the oncogenic potential of viral oncogenes, it is reasonable to suggest that the rapidity with which the neoplasm presents is a reflection of the fact that the virus encompasses all of the molecular requirements for conversion of a normal cell to a neoplastic cell and that this occurs shortly after integration of the viral genome into that of the host. Thus, in these few instances the answers to the questions are essentially the same.

However, at our present state of knowledge, such rapid induction of neoplasia is the exception rather than the rule. Both in experimental animals and in humans, induction of neoplasia by a variety of different agents—biological, chemical, or physical—usually requires prolonged periods (months or years) from the initial application of a carcinogenic agent to the development of cancer. A striking example of this phenomenon is the development of bronchogenic carcinoma following the chronic, excessive use of tobacco products, principally cigarettes (Doll and Peto 1981). In this example and in many others that are known, it is very unlikely that the answers to our questions are the same. Furthermore, when the answers are not the same, this affords at least two points of attack to control the disease. These approaches have been given the general terminology of prevention and therapy. The former is concerned with answers to question two, while the latter is related to question one.

Although the responses to the questions posed have been concerned with neoplasia in vivo, the questions may be similarly posed and in all likelihood answered through investigations of carcinogenesis in vitro, since the latter approach depends in the final analysis on the demonstration of malignant properties of the cell under conditions in vivo. Furthermore, since the entity under consideration in both questions is the same, i.e., cancer, a complete understanding of the answers to question two will encompass the answers to question one. For this reason, this overview will concern itself principally with the topic of this symposium, molecular carcinogenesis.

THE NATURAL HISTORY OF NEOPLASTIC DEVELOPMENT

As pointed out in this conference, it is possible to define distinct stages in the development of malignancy in mouse epidermis, both in vivo and in vitro (Slaga et al. 1987, Yuspa 1987), and in Syrian hamster embryo fibroblasts (Barrett et al. 1987). In addition, as pointed out by Drinkwater (1986), analogous stages may occur in mouse hepatic carcinogenesis, and other investigators have demonstrated the multistage nature of the development of a variety of neoplasms, both in animals and in humans (Pitot 1984). From these studies it is possible to characterize several of these stages that are common to all systems studied thus far. Such characteristics are listed briefly in Table 16.1.

The first stage, *initiation,* is irreversible, as judged by the possibility of an extended separation between the point of initiation and that of the beginning of the

Table 16.1. *Characteristics of the Stages in Neoplastic Development*

Initiation	Irreversible (spontaneous)
	Additive
	No threshold
Promotion	Reversible
	Environmentally modulated
	Maximal response
	Threshold
Progression	Irreversible
	Somatic aneuploidy
	Progressive karyotypic instability

second stage, promotion (Boutwell 1964, Peraino et al. 1977). However, for initiation to be effective, the process must occur in association with cellular replicative DNA synthesis and cell division (Ying et al. 1981, Warwick 1971, Borek and Sachs 1968). Although it has not been possible to identify single initiated cells unequivocally, their progeny can be identified either as papillomas in the skin (Boutwell 1964) or as foci of phenotypically altered cells in the liver (Emmelot and Scherer 1980). Similarly, foci of transformed cells occur in Syrian hamster embryo cell cultures treated with carcinogenic agents (Borek 1979, Barrett et al. 1987). All of these approaches allow some degree of quantitation of the initiating event. However, it should be noted that in all cases the clonal populations derived from initiated cells must be considered as developing during the stages of promotion or progression or both. Furthermore, initiation may occur fortuitously (spontaneously), as judged both in vivo and in vitro from the appearance of occasional focal lesions indistinguishable from clones derived from initiated cells (Schulte-Hermann et al. 1983) or the appearance of malignant neoplasms during the lifespan of an organism that has not been experimentally exposed to a carcinogen (Ward 1983). Finally, the process of initiation in skin (Verma and Boutwell 1980), liver (Emmelot and Scherer 1980), and other tissues (Peto et al. 1984, Maekawa et al. 1984) is a linear, additive, dose-related phenomenon and does not exhibit a readily measurable threshold.

The major characteristic of the stage of tumor *promotion* that distinguishes it from the stages of initiation and progression is that of its reversibility. Both in the epidermis (Stenbäck 1978, Iversen 1982) and the liver (Tatematsu et al. 1983, Glauert 1986), where quantitation of lesions occurring during promotion can be readily accomplished, the regression and reversibility of lesions demonstrate this principal characteristic of the stage of promotion. Furthermore, in models of multistage hepatocarcinogenesis in the rat, in which quantitation of initiated clones can be readily evaluated, the disappearance of such focal cell populations on removal of the promoting agent can be reversed by readministration of the promoting agent at a later date (Hendrich et al. 1986). These studies not only demonstrate the permanence of initiation but also the dependence of the phenotypically altered cells that develop from such initiated cells in the presence of the promoting agent. Such a phenomenon is analogous to the "dependent" neoplasms of endocrine tissues described by Furth (1968). The fact that environmental alterations including diet (Yang 1984), hormonal status (Lupulescu 1983), age (Van Duuren et al. 1978), and exogenous chemicals (Wattenberg 1985) can affect the stage of promotion has been well documented in a number of systems studied. Use of quantitative techniques has shown that, after initiation by a single dose of an initiating agent, promotion (even with increasing doses of the promoting agent) can ultimately lead only to a specific maximal response beyond which the promoting agent has no further effect until overt toxicity appears (Verma and Boutwell 1980, Goldsworthy et al. 1984). Such studies have also demonstrated the presence of a threshold or no-effect level of a promoting agent; this would be expected from the reversible nature of this stage of carcinogenesis.

The stage of *progression* is that irreversible stage in which benign or malignant neoplasms or both are characteristically seen. This stage has been defined as that stage of carcinogenesis exhibiting measurable (by recombinant DNA technology or similar methods) or morphologically discernible (karyotypic) changes in the structure of the cell genome (Pitot 1986). Thus, cells in the stage of progression exhibit somatic aneuploidy as viewed under the light microscope or by techniques of modern molecular biology. In this book we read that certain agents appear to act predominantly at this stage of neoplastic development (Slaga et al. 1987). Apparently concomitant with such chromosomal alterations comes an inherent progressive karyotypic instability. This was shown most strikingly by the earlier studies of Kraemer et al. (1972), who demonstrated the dramatic instability of karyotypes in established neoplasms. However, as has been pointed out by Nowell earlier (1986) and in this book (Nowell and Croce 1987), karyotypic instability is also a hallmark in the progression of human leukemias and lymphomas.

THE ROLE OF ONCOGENE EXPRESSION IN THE DEVELOPMENT OF CANCER

In this book there is considerable discussion of the genetics, the regulation of expression, and the structure of gene products of both viral and cellular oncogenes. The primary role of these genes and their products in malignant transformation by oncogenic retroviruses is undisputed. It is the v-*src* oncogene of the Rous sarcoma virus that in all likelihood is the principal cause of the dramatic cellular transformation to malignancy seen in vivo on infection with this virus. Similarly, other viruses, even those that are defective but that contain such oncogenes in the virion, induce a rapid, widespread, fatal malignant process. As pointed out earlier (vide supra), under these circumstances the molecular mechanisms of carcinogenesis appear to be rather straightforward. The role, if any, of proto-oncogene expression in multistage carcinogenesis has not been clarified. As has been pointed out in this symposium (Yuspa 1987) and as reported earlier by Balmain and his associates (1984), the c-Ha-*ras* is mutated very early during epidermal carcinogenesis in that more than 80% of papillomas exhibit this alteration when some chemical carcinogens are used to initiate and promote these lesions. Furthermore, both in epidermal and hepatocarcinogenesis (Balmain et al. 1984, Wiseman et al. 1986), in which such mutations in this gene occur after initiation with several different chemical carcinogens, the type of mutation is the one expected from a knowledge of the chemical actions of the carcinogen itself. However, the mere presence of a mutation does not, de facto, prove a central role for this alteration in initiation or other stages of carcinogenesis.

There is substantial evidence that many, if not most, neoplasms in the stage of progression either do possess mutated proto-oncogenes or express one or more normal proto-oncogenes at significantly higher levels than seen in the cell of origin (Spandidos 1985). Such "activation" of proto-oncogenes may result from specific translocations of chromosomal loci, especially regulatory elements (Nowell and Croce 1987), or from a variety of other mechanisms (Krontiris 1983), including the insertion of activated oncogenes directly into the fertilized egg (Adams et al. 1985). Furthermore, since the protein products of a number of viral and cellular oncogenes are either themselves growth factors or affect the mediation of growth factor signals (Goustin et al. 1986), it is reasonable to expect an increased function of growth signals during the stage of progression when neoplastic cells exhibit their greatest growth potential (Welch and Tomasovic 1985). As elegantly shown by the structural studies of the protein product of the viral and cellular Ha-*ras* gene, mutations themselves can lead to a major altered function of the gene product (McCormick et al. 1987) without a necessary and concomitant increase in the transcriptional rate of the gene. Even products of viral oncogenes from DNA oncogenic viruses may directly affect the phenotypic expression of proto-oncogenes (Cantley et al. 1987), which may in turn lead to alteration of metabolic pathways that have now been linked to an enzyme function directly related to a specific promoting agent, tetradecanoyl phorbol acetate (TPA) (Bell et al. 1987, Majerus et al. 1987). Thus, while proto-oncogene expression in multistage carcinogenesis at the present time seems to be predominantly associated with the stage of progression, there is evidence that such activation of proto-oncogenes may play a role much earlier in the development of cancer induced by chemical and physical agents (Balmain et al. 1984, Reynolds et al. 1986).

Proto-oncogene and growth factor expression also appear to play roles in specific regulatory mechanisms in vivo, such as rat liver regeneration (Fausto et al. 1987). Hepatocyte replication stimulated by removal of 70% of the liver results in dramatic increases in the transcription of several proto-oncogenes including c-*fos*, c-*myc*, and the p53 protein gene. Unlike the mouse (Reynolds et al. 1986), however, there is no evidence for consistent mutational activation of proto-oncogenes during multistage hepatocarcinogenesis in the rat, although evidence for transcriptional activation of such genes has been reported (Beer et al. 1986). In preliminary studies in our laboratory, Dr. Beer has demonstrated that the transcription of the c-*raf* oncogene in rat liver increases dramatically 20 hr after partial hepatectomy and that many primary hepatocellular carcinomas and neoplastic nodules investigated showed a similar increased transcription. However, in the neoplastic tissues such increased transcription of this proto-oncogene did not correlate with an increase in the transcription of the gene for H_4 histone, a hallmark of cellular proliferation, although such correlation was found following partial hepatectomy. Thus, cells in progression during multistage hepatocarcinogenesis in the rat may exhibit increased transcriptional rates of proto-oncogenes, but as yet no consistent pattern of such transcriptional alterations has been noted.

MOLECULAR MECHANISMS AND MULTISTAGE CARCINOGENESIS BY VARIOUS CARCINOGENS

The scheme of multistage carcinogenesis seen in Table 16.1 does not necessarily imply that cancer resulting from all possible carcinogenic agents will follow the multistage mechanism as outlined. Rather, as a result of this conference it has become clear that one or more of these stages may be absent or only rudimentary during carcinogenesis by various agents. An outline of these relationships is shown in Table 16.2.

Referring to the characteristics of the stages of multistage carcinogenesis listed in Table 16.1, it is possible to indicate those stages that are easily demonstrable in carcinogenesis by any one of the agents seen in Table 16.2. However, in some instances a slight overlap cannot be entirely ruled out. Carcinogenesis by viruses whose genetic information is integrated into the host genome at the time of initial infection bypasses the stages of initiation and promotion simply by our definition (Table 16.1; Pitot 1986). Any measurable addition of genetic information to the genome, such as following integration of viral genomes, would also place the cell in the stage of progression. The natural history of most such infections conforms to this, although some cases, such as the leukosis viruses, which do not possess viral oncogenes in their genome, may require prolonged periods before the appearance of malignancy (Hayward et al. 1981). Still, there is no evidence for a reversible stage under these circumstances. On the other hand, with viruses that infect cells, the resultant infection leading to an episomal relationship between the virus and the host genome may represent a stage analogous to promotion, as seen, for example, by the formation of papillomas in humans and animals (Fu et al. 1983, Gissmann 1984).

Table 16.2. *Stages Involved in Carcinogenesis by Various Agents*

Carcinogenesis	Stages
Viral	
With integration	Progression
Episomal	Promotion, progression
Chemical	
Low dose	Initiation, promotion, progression
High dose	Progression
Radiation	
Low dose	Initiation, promotion, progression
High dose	Progression
Genetic	
Spontaneous	Initiation, (promotion), progression
Induced	
Transfection	(Initiation), progression
Transgenic	Progression

However, once malignancy is apparent, the stage of progression is operative, and in the case of human genital papilloma virus infections, viral information becomes integrated into the host genome during this stage (Schwarz et al. 1985).

As emphasized in this symposium, chemical carcinogenesis induced by relatively low doses of carcinogenic agents and accompanied by minimal toxicity can be divided into the three stages of initiation, promotion, and progression. However, when very large, single, toxic doses of chemical carcinogens are given, many of the cells altered by the carcinogen may already have significant chromosomal damage and thus be in the stage of progression (Table 16.1). Similarly, radiation carcinogenesis with low doses can be associated with the same three stages, as has been previously reported from several laboratories (Fry et al. 1982, Holtzman et al. 1979, Curtis and Tilley 1972). Very high doses of ionizing radiation, however, usually result in significant chromosomal damage in most cells that remain viable, and thus the stage of progression is predominant.

In this book we have been introduced to the concept of genetic carcinogenesis, both spontaneous and induced. Dr. Dryja (1987) presented beautiful studies demonstrating the localization of a specific gene, in which a mutational change is probably directly related to the formation of retinoblastoma in the human. These studies, which developed from numerous earlier investigations (Knudson et al. 1975, Murphree and Benedict 1984), clearly demonstrated that all of the cells of the organism are initiated through a single recessive germ-line mutation, which by itself does not lead to the phenotypic expression of neoplasia. However, when there is an allelic mutation in the same gene, then a malignant neoplasm results directly from this homozygous state. Under these circumstances, according to our criteria in Table 16.1, the stages of initiation and progression may be easily identified, but no reversible stage of promotion has ever been noted. On the other hand, the induction of cancer in genetic conditions with high predispositions to various types of cancer such as xeroderma pigmentosa, multiple polyposis, and others may include a stage analogous to promotion by the criteria of Table 16.1 (Ponder 1980). Induced genetic carcinogenesis is a relatively new field; the process was first described in cell culture. A number of investigators (cf. Cooper and Lane 1984) have reported the "transformation" of cell lines by the transfection of DNA from neoplastic cells. However, the best example of a true transfectional carcinogenesis is perhaps that reported by Barrett and coworkers (1987) in primary cultures of Syrian hamster embryo cells, with transfection by two different viral oncogenes. In this instance one could argue that infection by only one of the genes leads to initiation, while that with the second results in progression in a manner similar to that seen with retinoblastoma, but involving two distinctly separate genetic loci. In this book we were introduced to the remarkable phenomenon of transgenic induction of neoplasia that may exhibit a high degree of tissue specificity (Adams et al. 1985) from tissue-specific regulatory signals introduced into the fertilized egg simultaneously. On the other hand, inoculation of viral oncogene constructs in the absence of such signals may lead to the induction of various types of neoplasms or other nonneoplastic pathologic conditions or both. Again, by the characteristics of Table 16.1, such neoplasms, which inevitably occur following the transgenic approach, should be considered as always in the stage of progression, by definition, but further studies may demonstrate that it is possible to delineate a stage analogous to promotion in such animals.

While there are still many questions to be answered in relation to the molecular mechanisms of carcinogenesis, an overall framework can be sketched that will allow investigators to relate their findings to other, very dissimilar models. This both extends our knowledge of the details of this sketch and presents numerous potential experiments to be carried out in the future.

REFERENCES

Adams JM, Harris AW, Pinkert CA, et al. 1985. The c-*myc* oncogene driven by immunoglobulin enhancers induces lymphoid malignancy in transgenic mice. Nature 318: 533–538.

Balmain A, Sauerborn R, Ramsden M, et al. 1984. Oncogene activation at different stages of chemical carcinogenesis in mouse skin. *In* Genetic Variability in Responses to Chemical Exposure. Cold Spring Harbor Laboratory, Cold Spring Harbor, New York.

Barrett JC, Oshimura M, Koi M. 1987. Role of oncogenes and tumor-suppressor genes in a multistep model of carcinogenesis. Symp Fundam Cancer Res 39:45–56.

Beard JW. 1980. Biology of avian oncornaviruses. *In* Klein G, ed., Viral Oncology. Raven Press, New York, pp. 55–87.

Beer DG, Schwarz M, Sawada N, Pitot HC. 1986. Expression of H-*ras* and c-*myc* protooncogenes in isolated gamma-glutamyl transpeptidase-positive rat hepatocytes and in hepatocellular carcinomas induced by diethylnitrosamine. Cancer Res 46:2435–2441.

Bell RM, Hannun YA, Loomis CR. 1987. Mechanism of regulation of protein kinase C by lipid second messengers. Symp Fundam Cancer Res 39:145–156.

Borek C. 1979. Malignant transformation *in vitro:* Criteria, biological markers, and application in environmental screening of carcinogens. Radiat Res 79:209–232.

Borek C, Sachs L. 1968. The number of cell generations required to fix the transformed state in x-ray-induced transformation. Proc Natl Acad Sci USA 59:83–85.

Boutwell RK. 1964. Some biological aspects of skin carcinogenesis. Progr Exp Tumor Res 4:207–250.

Cantley LC, Whitman M, Kaplan DR, et al. Phosphatidylinositol kinases and cell transformation. Symp Fundam Cancer Res 39:165–172.

Cooper GM, Lane MA. 1984. Cellular transforming genes and oncogenesis. Biochim Biophys Acta 738:9–20.

Curtis HJ, Tilley J. 1972. The role of mutations in liver tumor induction in mice. Radiat Res 50:539–542.

Doll R, Peto R. 1981. The causes of cancer. Oxford University Press, Oxford.

Drinkwater NR, Ginsler JJ. 1986. Genetic control of hepatocarcinogenesis in C57BL/6J and C3H/HeJ inbred mice. Carcinogenesis 7:1701–1707.

Dryja TP, Friend S, Weinberg RA. 1987. Genetic sequences that predispose to retinoblastoma and osteosarcoma. Symp Fundam Cancer Res 39:115–119.

Emmelot P, Scherer E. 1980. The first relevant cell stage in rat liver carcinogenesis. A quantitative approach. Biochim Biophys Acta 605:247–304.

Fausto N, Mead JE, Braun L, et al. 1987. Proto-oncogene expression and growth factors during liver regeneration. Symp Fundam Cancer Res 39:69–86.

Fry RJM, Ley RD, Grube D, Staffeldt E. 1982. Studies on the multistage nature of radiation carcinogenesis. Carcinogenesis 7:155–165.

Fu YS, Braun L, Shah KV, Lawrence WD, Robboy, SJ. 1983. Histologic, nuclear DNA, and human papillomavirus. Studies of cervical condylomas. Cancer 52:1705–1711.

Furth J. 1968. Hormones and neoplasia. Third Internatl Symposium on Cancer and Aging. Nordiska Bokhaudelus Förlag, Stockholm, pp. 131–151.

Gissman L. 1984. Papillomaviruses and their association with cancer in animals and in man. Cancer Surveys 3:161–181.

Glauert HP, Schwarz M, Pitot HC. 1986. The phenotypic stability of altered hepatic foci: Effect of the short-term withdrawal of phenobarbital and of the long-term feeding of purified diets after the withdrawal of phenobarbital. Carcinogenesis 7:117–121.

Goldsworthy T, Campbell HA, Pitot HC. 1984. The natural history and dose-response characteristics of enzyme-altered foci in rat liver following phenobarbital and diethylnitrosamine administration. Carcinogenesis 5:67–71.

Goustin AS, Leof EB, Shipley GD, Moses HL. 1986. Growth factors and cancer. Cancer Res 46:1015–1029.

Hayward WS, Neel BG, Astrin SM. 1981. Activation of a cellular *onc* gene by promoter insertion in ALV-induced lymphoid leukosis. Nature 290:475–480.

Hendrich S, Glauert HP, Pitot HC. 1986. The phenotypic stability of altered hepatic foci: Effects of withdrawal and subsequent readministration of phenobarbital. Carcinogenesis 7:2041–2045.

Holtzman S, Stone JP, Shellabarger CJ. 1979. Synergism of diethylstilbestrol and radiation in mammary carcinogenesis in female F344 rats. JNCI 63:1071–1074.

Iversen OH. 1982. Hairless mouse skin in two-stage chemical carcinogenesis. Virchows Arch 38:263–272.

Knudson AG Jr, Hethcote HW, Brown BW. 1975. Mutation and childhood cancer: A probabilistic model for the incidence of retinoblastoma. Proc Natl Acad Sci USA 72:5116–5120.

Kraemer PM, Deaven LL, Crissman HA, VanDilla MA. 1972. DNA constancy despite variability in chromosome number. *In* DuPraw EJ, ed., Advances in Cell and Molecular Biology, vol. 2. Academic Press, New York, pp. 47–108.

Krontiris TG. 1983. The emerging genetics of human cancer. N Engl J Med 309:404–409.

Lupulescu A. 1983. Glucagon control of carcinogenesis. Endocrinology 113:527–534.

Maekawa A, Ogiu T, Matsuoka C, et al. 1984. Carcinogenicity of low doses of N-ethyl-N-nitrosourea in F344 rats, a dose-response study. Gann 75:117–125.

Majerus P, Connolly TM, Ross TS, Ishii H, Deckmyn H. 1987. The role of phosphoinositides in cell physiology. Symp Fundam Cancer Res 39:157–163.

McCormick F, Levenson C, Cole G, Innis M, Clark R. 1987. Genetic and biochemical analysis of *ras* p21 structure. Symp Fundam Cancer Res 39:137–142.

Murphree AL, Benedict WF. 1984. Retinoblastoma: Clues to human oncogenesis. Science 223:1028–1033.

Nowell PC. 1986. Mechanisms of tumor progression. Cancer Res 46:2203–2207.

Nowell PC, Croce CM. 1987. Chromosomal approaches to the molecular basis of neoplasia. Symp Fundam Cancer Res 39:17–29.

Peraino C, Fry RJM, Staffeldt E. 1977. Effects of varying the onset and duration of exposure to phenobarbital on its enhancement of 2-acetylamino-fluorene-induced hepatic tumorigenesis. Cancer Res 37:3623–3627.

Peto R, Gray R, Brantom P, Grasso P. 1984. Nitrosamine carcinogenesis in 5120 rodents: Chronic administration of sixteen different concentrations of NDEA, NDMA, NPYR and NPIP in the water of 4440 inbred rats, with parallel studies on NDEA alone of the effect of age of starting (3, 6 or 20 weeks) and of species (rats, mice or hamsters). *In* O'Neill IK, Von Borstel RC, Miller CT, Long J, Bartsch H, eds., N-Nitroso Compounds: Occurrence, Biological Effects and Relevance to Human Cancer. International Agency for Research on Cancer, Lyon, pp. 627–665.

Pitot HC. 1986. Fundamentals of Oncology, Third Edition. Marcel Dekker, Inc., New York, p. 167.

Pitot HC. 1984. Triggering the cellular change to neoplasia. J Urol 23(Suppl.):9–17.

Ponder BAJ. 1980. Genetics and cancer. Biochim Biophys Acta 605:369–410.

Reynolds SH, Stowers SJ, Maranpot RR, Anderson MW, Aaronson SA. 1986. Detection and identification of activated oncogenes in spontaneously occurring benign and malignant hepatocellular tumors of the B6C3F1 mouse. Proc Natl Acad Sci USA 83:33–37.

Schulte-Hermann R, Timmermann-Trosiener I, Schuppler J. 1983. Promotion of spontaneous preneoplastic cells in rat liver as a possible explanation of tumor production by nonmutagenic compounds. Cancer Res 43:839–844.

Schwarz E, Freese UK, Gissmann L, et al. 1985. Structure and transcription of human papillomavirus sequences in cervical carcinoma cells. Nature 314:111–114.

Slaga TJ, O'Connell J, Rotstein J, et al. 1987. Critical genetic determinants and molecular events in multistage skin carcinogenesis. Symp Fundam Cancer Res 39:31–44.

Spandidos DA. 1985. Mechanism of carcinogenesis: The role of oncogenes, transcriptional enhancers and growth factors. Anticancer Res 5:485–498.

Stenbäck F. 1978. Tumor persistence and regression in skin carcinogenesis. Z Krebsforsch 91:249–259.

Tatematsu M, Nagamine Y, Farber E. 1983. Redifferentiation as a basis for remodeling of carcinogen-induced hepatocyte nodules to normal appearing liver. Cancer Res 43:5049–5056.

Van Duuren BL, Smith AC, Melchionne SM. 1978. Effect of aging in two-stage carcinogenesis on mouse skin with phorbol myristate acetate as promoting agent. Cancer Res 38:865–866.

Verma AJ, Boutwell RK. 1980. Effects of dose and duration of treatment with the tumor-promoting agent, 12-0-tetradecanoylphorbol-13-acetate on mouse skin carcinogenesis. Carcinogenesis 1:271–276.

Ward JM 1983. Background data and variations in tumor rates of control rats and mice. Prog Exp Tumor Res 26:241–258.

Warwick GP. 1971. Effect of the cell cycle on carcinogenesis. Fed Proc 30:1760–1765.

Wattenberg LW. 1985. Chemoprevention of cancer. Cancer Res 45:1–8.

Welch DR, Tomasovic SP. 1985. Implications of tumor progression on clinical oncology. Clin Exp Metastasis 3:151–188.

Wiseman RW, Stowers SJ, Miller EC, Anderson MW, Miller JA. 1986. Activating mutations of the c-Ha-*ras* protooncogene in chemically induced hepatomas of the male B6C3F$_1$ mouse. Proc Natl Acad Sci USA 83:5825–5829.

Yang CS. 1984. Modification of carcinogenesis by dietary and nutritional factors. *In* Chu EHY, Generoso WM, eds., Environmental Mutagenesis, Carcinogenesis, and Teratogenesis. Plenum Press, New York, pp. 465–485.

Ying TS, Sarma DSR, Farber E. 1981. Role of acute hepatic necrosis in the induction of early steps in liver carcinogenesis by diethylnitrosamine. Cancer Res 41:2096–2102.

Yuspa SH. 1987. Cellular and molecular mechanisms of carcinogenesis in lining epithelia. Symp Fundam Cancer Res 39:3–15.

Contributors

Claudio M. Aldaz
The University of Texas System Cancer
  Center
Science Park—Research Division
Smithville, TX 78957

J. Carl Barrett
Environmental Carcinogenesis Group
National Institute of Environmental Health
  Sciences
Research Triangle Park, NC 27709

Graeme I. Bell
Howard Hughes Medical Institute
Department of Biochemistry and Molecular
  Biology
University of Chicago
Chicago, IL 60637

Robert M. Bell
Department of Biochemistry
Duke University Medical Center
Durham, NC 27710

Lundy Braun
Department of Pathology and Laboratory
  Medicine
Brown University
Providence, RI 02912

Lewis C. Cantley
Department of Physiology
Tufts University School of Medicine
Boston, MA 02111

Suresh Chahwala
Department of Physiology
Tufts University School of Medicine
Boston, MA 02111

Robin Clark
Department of Molecular Biology
Cetus Corporation
Emeryville, CA 94608

Georgette Cole
Department of Microbial Genetics
Cetus Corporation
Emeryville, CA 94608

Thomas M. Connolly
Division of Hematology-Oncology
Washington University School of Medicine
St. Louis, MO 63110

Claudio J. Conti
The University of Texas System Cancer
  Center
Science Park—Research Division
Smithville, TX 78957

Carlo Croce
The Wistar Institute of Anatomy and Biology
Philadelphia, PA 19104

Hans Deckmyn
Divison of Hematology-Oncology
Washington University School of Medicine
St. Louis, MO 63110

Thaddeus P. Dryja
Massachusetts Eye and Ear Infirmary and
  Harvard Medical School
Boston, MA 02115

Gerde Endemann
Department of Physiology
Tufts University School of Medicine
Boston, MA 02111

Nelson Fausto
Department of Pathology and Laboratory
   Medicine
Brown University
Providence, RI 02912

Laurie Fleischman
Department of Physiology
Tufts University School of Medicine
Boston, MA 02111

Stephen Friend
Whitehead Institute for Biomedical Research
   and Massachusetts Institute of Technology
Cambridge, MA 02142

Lillian Glazer
Department of Virology
The Weizmann Institute of Science
Rehovot 76100, Israel

Dorit S. Ginsberg
Department of Virology
The Weizmann Institute of Science
Rehovot 76100, Israel

Michele Goyette
Department of Pathology and Laboratory
   Medicine
Brown University
Providence, RI 02912

Yusuf A. Hannun
Departments of Biochemistry and Medicine
Duke University Medical Center
Durham, NC 27710

Steven K. Hanks
The Salk Institute
San Diego, CA 92138

Gerard M. Housey
Comprehensive Cancer Center and Institute
   of Cancer Research
Columbia University College of Physicians
   and Surgeons
New York, NY 10032

Wendy Hsiao
Comprehensive Cancer Center and Institute
   of Cancer Research
Columbia University College of Physicians
   and Surgeons
New York, NY 10032

Michael Innis
Department of Microbial Genetics
Cetus Corporation
Emeryville, CA 94608

Hidemi Ishii
Division of Hematology-Oncology
Washington University School of Medicine
St. Louis, MO 63110

Rudolf Jaenisch
Whitehead Institute for Biomedical Research
Cambridge, MA 02142

Mark D. Johnson
Comprehensive Cancer Center and Institute
   of Cancer Research
Columbia University College of Physicians
   and Surgeons
New York, NY 10032

David R. Kaplan
Laboratory of Neoplastic Disease
   Mechanisms
Dana-Farber Cancer Institute and the
   Department of Pathology
Harvard Medical School
Boston, MA 02115

Paul Kirschmeier
Comprehensive Cancer Center and Institute
   of Cancer Research
Columbia University College of Physicians
   and Surgeons
New York, NY 10032

Minoru Koi
Environmental Carcinogenesis Group
National Institute of Environmental Health
   Sciences
Research Triangle Park, NC 27709

Corey Levenson
Department of Chemistry
Cetus Corporation
Emeryville, CA 94608

Carson R. Loomis
Department of Biochemistry
Duke University Medical Center
Durham, NC 27710

Philip W. Majerus
Division of Hematology-Oncology
Washington University School of Medicine
St. Louis, MO 63110

Frank McCormick
Department of Molecular Biology
Cetus Corporation
Emeryville, CA 94608

Janet E. Mead
Department of Pathology and Laboratory
    Medicine
Brown University
Providence, RI 02912

Richard L. Mitchell
California Biotechnology, Inc.
Mountain View, CA 94043

Rebecca Morris
The University of Texas System Cancer
    Center
Science Park—Research Division
Smithville, TX 78957

Eva J. Neer
Cardiovascular Division
Brigham and Women's Hospital and Harvard
    Medical School
Boston, MA 02115

Peter C. Nowell
Department of Pathology and Laboratory
    Medicine
University of Pennsylvania Medical School
Philadelphia, PA 19104

Catherine A. O'Brian
Comprehensive Cancer Center and Institute
    of Cancer Research
Columbia University College of Physicians
    and Surgeons
New York, NY 10032

John O'Connell
The University of Texas System Cancer
    Center
Science Park—Research Division
Smithville, TX 78957

Mitsuo Oshimura
Environmental Carcinogenesis Group
National Institute of Environmental Health
    Sciences
Research Triangle Park, NC 27709

Marilyn Panzica
Department of Pathology and Laboratory
    Medicine
Brown University
Providence, RI 02912

George Patskan
The University of Texas System Cancer
    Center
Science Park—Research Division
Smithville, TX 78957

Henry C. Pitot
McArdle Laboratory for Cancer Research
    and the Departments of Oncology and
    Pathology
The Medical School
University of Wisconsin
Madison, WI 53706

Thomas M. Roberts
Laboratory of Neoplastic Disease
    Mechanisms
Dana-Farber Cancer Institute
Harvard Medical School
Boston, MA 02115

Theodora S. Ross
Division of Hematology-Oncology
Washington University School of Medicine
St. Louis, MO 63110

Joel Rotstein
The University of Texas System Cancer
    Center
Science Park—Research Division
Smithville, TX 78957

Brian S. Schaffhausen
Department of Biochemistry
Tufts University School of Medicine
Boston, MA 02111

Eyal D. Schejter
Department of Virology
The Weizmann Institute of Science
Rehovot 76100, Israel

Daniel Segal
Department of Neurobiology
The Weizmann Institute of Science
Rehovot 76100, Israel

Peter R. Shank
Section of Molecular Cellular and Develop-
    mental Biology
Brown University
Providence, RI 02912

Ben-Zion Shilo
Department of Virology
The Weizmann Institute of Science
Rehovot 76100, Israel

Thomas J. Slaga
The University of Texas System Cancer
    Center
Science Park—Research Division
Smithville, TX 78957

Philippe Soriano
Whitehead Institute for Biomedical Research
Cambridge, MA 02142

Nancy L. Thompson
Laboratory of Chemoprevention
National Cancer Institute
Bethesda, MD 20892

Inder M. Verma
The Salk Institute
San Diego, CA 92138

Robert A. Weinberg
Whitehead Institute for Biomedical Research
    and Massachusetts Institute of Technology
Cambridge, MA 02142

I. Bernard Weinstein
Comprehensive Cancer Center and Institute
    of Cancer Research
Columbia University College of Physicians
    and Surgeons
New York, NY 10032

Malcolm Whitman
Department of Physiology
Tufts University School of Medicine
Boston, MA 02111

Stuart H. Yuspa
Laboratory of Cellular Carcinogenesis and
    Tumor Promotion
National Cancer Institute
Bethesda, MD 20892

Index